Eduardo Álvarez

Evolution of Dentition

Eduardo Álvarez

Evolution of Dentition

Update

ScienciaScripts

Imprint

Any brand names and product names mentioned in this book are subject to trademark, brand or patent protection and are trademarks or registered trademarks of their respective holders. The use of brand names, product names, common names, trade names, product descriptions etc. even without a particular marking in this work is in no way to be construed to mean that such names may be regarded as unrestricted in respect of trademark and brand protection legislation and could thus be used by anyone.

Cover image: www.ingimage.com

This book is a translation from the original published under ISBN 978-620-2-14914-3.

Publisher:
Sciencia Scripts
is a trademark of
Dodo Books Indian Ocean Ltd. and OmniScriptum S.R.L publishing group

120 High Road, East Finchley, London, N2 9ED, United Kingdom
Str. Armeneasca 28/1, office 1, Chisinau MD-2012, Republic of Moldova, Europe
Printed at: see last page
ISBN: 978-620-7-88829-0

Contents

Authors:
Dr. Estefanía Castro.
Dr. Eduardo Alvarez
Dr. Nedy Calderón.
Dr. Maria Angelica Cereceda.

"Evolution of Dentition. Update" Self-instruction Manual. Santiago. Universidad de Chile, Facultad de Odontología, Departamento del niño y ortopedia dentomaxilar, Área de Ortodoncia y Ortopedia dentomaxilar. 2015.

INTRODUCTION

Knowledge of the evolution of the dentition is of fundamental importance for those involved in dentistry. Teeth begin their formation inside the jaws in intrauterine life, forming the primary dentition and later the permanent dentition.

Both dentitions, primary and permanent, are equally important and their harmonious development will be key in maintaining adequate dento-maxillo-facial conditions, in turn influencing the functional and social development of the individual.

Knowledge of the characteristics of the development of the dentition under normal conditions will allow the dentist to detect dentition alterations early, in order to intervene when necessary and thus prevent the development of various dentomaxillary anomalies, which will be detrimental to the patient, as well as to understand the possible causes and take appropriate decisions when a dentomaxillary anomaly is already in place.

On the other hand, knowledge of the development of the dentition will enable the dentist to guide parents and/or patients with common questions during the development of teeth, some of which are quite frequent.

This manual is addressed to all those who are interested in knowing how the development of both dentitions takes place under normal conditions and in harmonious relationship with the rest of the creaneofacial structures, especially to dental students and all those who are involved in this area.

The manual consists of three chapters: Primary Dentition, Mixed Dentition First Phase and Mixed Dentition Second Phase, each of which is made up of units, which in turn are made up of their respective sub-units. At the beginning of each unit you will find the unit objectives, which you will want to achieve. At the end of each unit you will find a test that you will have to develop, which you will be able to revise with the solutions that will appear below. Each chapter has its respective bibliographical references, which you will be able to consult once you have finished each one of them. Finally, after the three chapters there is a final test with which you will be able to self-evaluate your learning in relation to the manual.

You will be able to organise your time and review each content as many times as you consider convenient. The idea is that this manual will help you to understand the main characteristics of the evolution of the dentition, so that you will be the one to organise your study, adapting it as you see fit.

CHAPTER 1

PRIMARY DENTITION
I UNIT: PRENATAL STAGE

> **Objectives**
> *By the end of this unit you will be able to explain:*
> I. *The formation of the main facial structures in the prenatal stage.*
> II. *The relationships adopted by the jaws at this stage.*
> III. *The formation of teeth in intrauterine life (odontogenesis).*
> IV. *The location of the teeth within the jaws, prior to birth.*

1) DEVELOPMENT OF FACIAL STRUCTURES

Towards the end of the 4th[0] week of intrauterine life, the facial processes or prominences appear (Fig. 1), which consist mainly of mesenchyme from the neural crest and are formed by the first pair of pharyngeal arches, these are :

- **Prominence of the upper jaw:** there are two of them, located dorsal to the first pharyngeal arch and lateral to the stomodeum.
- **Lower maxillary prominences:** two in number, located caudal to the stomodeum
- **Frontonasal prominence:** elevation cranial to the stomodeum. On both sides of it, there are fatty deposits called *nasal placodes 1*.

Nasal cavities: at $5°$ week the *nasal placodes* invaginate and form the *nasal fossae,* in this process creating a ridge of tissue that surrounds the fossae and forms the *lateral and* medial *nasal prominences*. At $6°$ week, the nasal fossae deepen, due to the growth of the nasal prominences that form the nasal cavities.

They are surrounded by and enter the underlying mesenchyme. The *bucconasal membrane* that separated the fossae from the primitive oral cavity is broken and they flow into the nasal cavity through the primitive choanae, which will later be located at the junction of the nasal oral cavity with the pharynx.

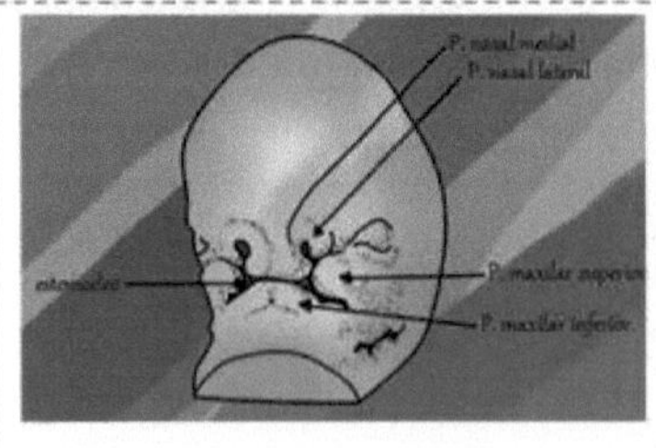

Fig. 1, Embrión de seis semanas y media. (Moyers 1992). Dibujado Por Castro E.

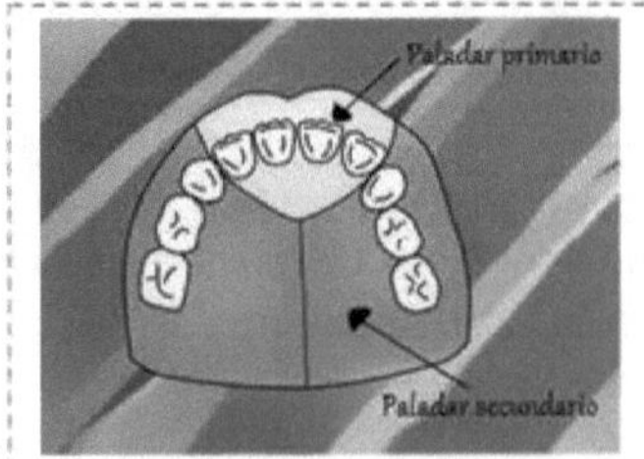

Fig. 2, Paladar definitivo. (Langman 2010). Dibujado por Castro E.

Upper lip: Forms within two weeks after the formation of the nostrils, from the junction of the *medial nasal prominences* and the *upper maxillary prominences.*

Intermaxillary segment: Corresponds to the structures formed by the junction of the *medial nasal prominences*. It is formed by: a *labial component,* an *upper maxillary component* leading to the four incisors, and a *palatine component* forming the **primary or primitive palate**[2].

Secondary palate: It is formed from the *palatine ridges,* which are ridge-shaped protuberances of the upper maxillary processes, which appear in the 6th° week of development and towards the 7th° week ascend, horizontalising and joining together to form the *secondary palate.* Towards the front they unite with the *primary palate to form* the *definitive palate* (Fig. 2), leaving as a vestige of this the *palatine foramen.*

Lower lip and Mandible: Formed from the fusion of the *lower jaw prominences.*

Tongue formation. It is formed by the fusion of two lingual protrusions that appear around 4° week of intrauterine life, giving rise to the anterior two thirds or body of the tongue. The mucosa covering the body of the tongue comes from the first pharyngeal arch, which is why this area is innervated by the inferior maxillary branch of the trigeminal nerve. The body of the tongue is separated posteriorly by the terminal sulcus, which is V-shaped.

The posterior portion of the tongue originates from the second, third and part of the fourth pharyngeal arch and in the adult the sensory innervation of this area comes from the glossopharyngeal nerve, probably because the part corresponding to the third pharyngeal arch grew more than that corresponding to the second arch. The most posterior portion of the tongue is innervated by the superior laryngeal nerve from the fourth pharyngeal arch 2.

2) RELATIONS BETWEEN THE JAWS DURING THE PRENATAL PERIOD.

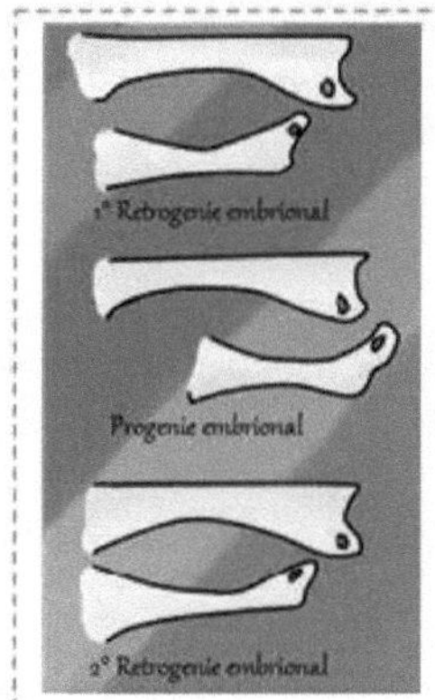

Fig. 3, Maxillary relations in the prenatal period. (Bruhn 1944). Drawn by Castro E.

Prior to birth, the relationship between the upper jaw and the mandible undergoes variations (Fig. 3), as follows:

❖ **First embryonic retrogenesis:** This relationship can be observed during the *tenth week* of intrauterine life and refers to the mandible being in a distal position to the upper jaw.

❖ **Embryonic progeny:** Observed between the *eleventh and twelfth week* of intrauterine life. After the union of the palatine processes, the mandible is located mesial to the maxilla. upper 3'.

❖ **Second embryonic retrogenesis:** This relationship can be found from the *twelfth week* of intrauterine life and is *maintained until birth,* where the mandible again acquires a distant position with respect to the upper jaw.

3) DEVELOPMENT OF THE PRIMARY TEETH. ODONTOGENESIS.

By the 6th week of intrauterine life, from the basal layer of the epithelial lining of the oral cavity, the **dental lamina** forms, a c-shaped structure that will be located along the jaws.

After a short time, 10 buds per jawbone will appear on the dental lamina, called **dental buds.** Later, due to the invagination of their surface, the buds will acquire a new shape called: **Fasedecasquete.**

The cap is formed by an *external and internal dental* epithelium *and a stellate reticulum centre.* The mesenchyme in the cleft forms the **dental papilla.**

Due to its growth and the deepening of its cleft, the cap acquires a new morphology, giving rise to a new phase called the **Bell Phase,** after the shape it acquires. At this stage, the cells of the papilla will differentiate into **odontoblasts**, dentine-producing cells, which after the formation of dentine will leave a layer called the *dentine process.* The remaining cells of the papilla will form the **pulp.** The cells of the inner epithelium will differentiate into **ameloblasts,** enamel-producing cells. Once the enamel has been produced, a temporary membrane called **cutuladental^** will remain on top of the enamel.

Root formation begins when the dental epithelial layers penetrate the mesenchyme and form the **root epithelial layer.** The cells of the dental papilla will deposit layers of dentine that continue into the crown, leaving a canal inside through which blood vessels and nerves will pass.

Mesenchymal cells located outside the tooth and in contact with dentine will differentiate into **cementoblasts** (cementum-producing cells), and outside the tooth the mesenchymal cells will give rise to the **periodontal igament (**Fig 5).

The activity of the dental lamina is not continuous, as it is alternated by moments of rest, initially forming the germs of the primary teeth, and after a proliferation of the lamina towards the lingual or palate, the permanent germs are formed (Fig. 4). The activity of the lamina can be summarised in the following periods: the formation of the primary germs is from six months of intrauterine life or one and a half to two months. The permanent germs of permanent premolars, incisors and canines are formed from 4° months of intrauterine life to 10 months of age, while the germs of the second and third permanent molars are formed from 10 months of age to 5 years 5.

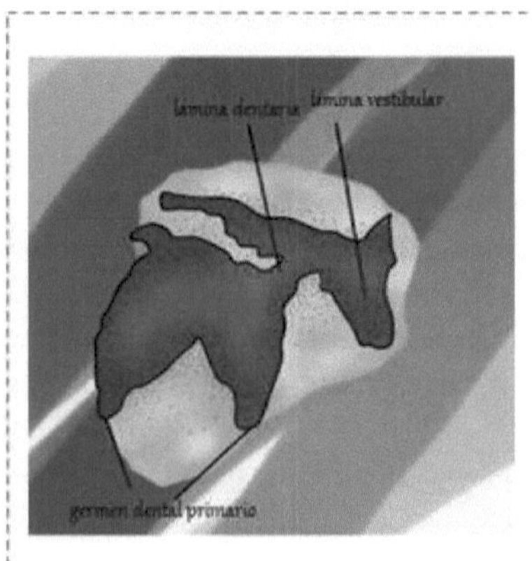

Fig. 4, Primary tooth germ (Montenegro). Drawn

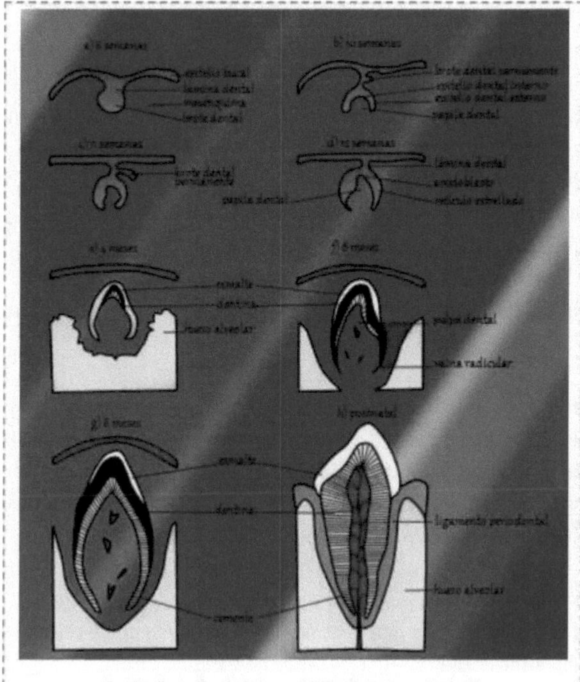

Fig. 5, Odontogénesis. (Moyers 1992). Dibujado por Castro E.

4) LOCATION OF PRIMARY TEETH WITHIN THE JAWS IN THE PRENATAL PERIOD

The germs are not positioned in an orderly fashion as they penetrate the mesenchyme, nor do they emerge in a completely perpendicular direction.

Towards the *seventh month of intrauterine life* there is a crowding in both jaws due to primitive Intramesenchymal implantation defects, to which is added a volumetric problem, as the joint growth of the germs is greater than that of the jaws, generating a crowding that conserves a certain morphological pattern:

1. The incisors are crowded with the lateral incisors placed lingually; the central incisors are more often in a regular position.

2. The molars overlap and overlap with different levels of vertical θ-implantation.

TEST OF THE FIRST UNIT

1. Which processes originate from the first pair of pharyngeal arches?
a) 1 upper maxillary process, 2 lower maxillary processes and 2 frontonasal processes
b) 1 nasal placode, 2 lateral nasal prominences and 2 medial nasal prominences
c) 2 upper maxillary processes ,2 lower maxillary processes and 1 frontonasal process
d) 1 stomodeum, 2 nasal placodes, 2 maxillary maxillary processes.

2. From which structures is the upper lip formed?
a) Junction of the intermaxillary segment with the frontonasal process
b) Union of the medial nasal prominences with the upper maxillary prominences
c) Junction of the intermaxillary segment with the palatine ridges
d) Union of the lateral nasal prominences with the upper maxillary prominences.

3. Which of the components of the intermaxillary segment contains the four upper incisors?
a) Maxillary-inferior component
b) Palatal component
c) Lip component
(d) Uppermaxillary component

4. From which structures does the secondary palate form?
a) Apartirdecrestaspalatinas
b) From the lower maxillary prominences
c) From the first and second gill arch onwards
d) Apart from the nasal plates.

5. From the union of which structures is the definitive palate formed?
a) attachment of the labial component to the palatal component
b) attachment of the palatal component to the primary palate.
c) junction of the primitive palate with the secondary palate.
d) junction of the primary palate with the primitive palate.

6. Between which weeks can the second embryonic retrogeny be found?
a) Between the eleventh and twelfth week of intrauterine life.
b) Between the tenth and twelfth week of intrauterine life.
c) Between the eleventh week of intrauterine life until birth.
d) Between the twelfth week of intrauterine life until birth.

7.   In what order do the stages of odontogenesis take place?

a)   Dental plate - dental buds - cap phase - bell phase.

b)   Dental buds - bell phase - cap phase - dental lamina.

c)   Tooth buds - cap stage - bell stage.

d)   Dental plate - dental buds - bell phase - cap phase.

8.   In which weeks does the formation of tooth germs begin in the primary and permanent dentition?

a) $4°$ and $6°$ week of intrauterine life.

b) $4°$ week and $6°$ month of intrauterine life.

c) $6°$ week and $4°$ month of intrauterine life.

d)   4 and 6^{00} month of intrauterine life.

9.   Why does crowding of the dental germs occur during the $7°$ month of intrauterine life?

a)   Because the size of the jaws is much larger in relation to the size of the dental germs and because of their poor implantation.

Intramesenchymatous

b)   Due to primitive defects of intramesenchymatous implantation of the germs and because the size of the jaws is smaller in relation to the size of the dental germs.

c)   Because the molars are overlapping and overlapping at different levels of implantation.

d)   Because the germs of the permanent teeth are located lingually and palatally to the primary teeth.

SOLUTIONS TO THE FIRST UNIT TEST

1.   c) 2 upper maxillary processes ,2 lower maxillary processes and 1 frontonasal process

2.   (b) junction of the medial nasal prominences with the maxillary upper prominences

3.   d)Upper jaw component

4.   (a) From palatine ridges

5.   c) By the junction of the primitive palate with the secondary palate.

6.   (d) Between the twelfth week of intrauterine life until birth.

7.   (a) Dental plate - dental buds - cap phase - bell phase.

8.   c) $6°$ week and $4°$ month of intrauterine life.

9.   b) Due to primitive defects in the intramesenchymatous implantation of the germs and because the size of the jaws is smaller in relation to the size of the dental germs.

UNIT II: PRIMARY DENTITION FROM OALOSS MONTHS OF AGE.

Objectives
By the end of this unit you will be able to explain:
I.   The anatomical features of the lips and oral cavity during the period from losO to 5 months.
II.   The characteristics and relationships between the jaws in this period.
III.   What positions do the germs of the teeth adopt between the ages of 0-5 months?
IV.   What is the level of calcification of teeth at birth.
V.   How it develops and the importance of breastfeeding.

1. ANATOMICAL CHARACTERISTICS OF THE LIPS AND ORAL CAVITY OF THE INFANT BETWEEN THE AGES OF FIVE MONTHS AND FIVE MONTHS.

In the first months of life, the baby's feeding is exclusively liquid and will be carried out through breastfeeding, so the newborn's mouth has special characteristics that will allow it to fulfil this function, among them we find:

Lips: They have radial prominences in red called **suction rims** (Fig. 5), whose function is to seal the θ areola.

Alveolar processes: they are not smooth, they are covered with ridges and furrows, on their external sides they have eminences corresponding to the germs of the incisors and canines, they often have an incurvation so that when they close they do not contact the anterior sector^.

In the upper arch the alveolar ridge is wide and flattened, and in its anterior part there is an **incisor platform** whose size varies between 8 to 10 mm, while in the lower arch the alveolar ridge is narrow and sharp^.

Gums: firm, their shape is determined in intrauterine life, they are horseshoe-shaped, in sagittal view the lower gum is seen behind the upper gum and both extend labially and buccally beyond the alveolar bone^.

Gingival cushions: structures that cover the alveolar processes at birth, which are soon segmented to indicate the sites of the developing teeth.

Gingival membrane or fibrous cord of Robin and Magitot: This is a mucous fold in the shape of a comb, formed by small papillary eminences in the shape of a fringe, it is highly vascularised and is erectile, protruding 1 mm θ. It is observed from occlusal over the corresponding areas where incisors and canines will erupt, which disappears during the period of dental eruption and whose function is to facilitate swallowing during suckling θ (Fig. 6).

Palate: It is flat and is limited by the **lateral palatine weatherstrips,** which allow the nipple and areola to be encased in the oral cavity, collaborating with the hermetic seal ∧ The palatine weatherstrips form the **palatal concavity** which serves as a cradle for the maternal nipple. It also has **transverse palatal folds,** which are more pronounced in the newborn than in the child and adult, there are 4 to 5 pairs that increase the rubbing of the anterior region allowing the nipple to be supported in the pressure phase θ (Fig. 7).

Cheeks: has the presence of the **cheek fat ball,** which is a conglomerate of fat located between the buccinator and the masseter, which will serve as a muscular cushion during suckling ∧

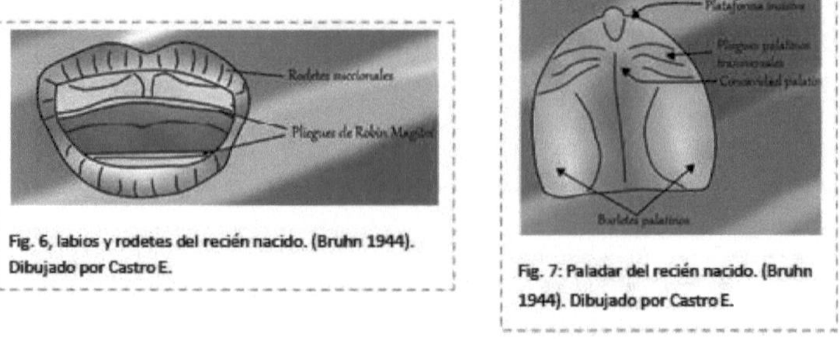

Fig. 6, labios y rodetes del recién nacido. (Bruhn 1944). Dibujado por Castro E.

Fig. 7: Paladar del recién nacido. (Bruhn 1944). Dibujado por Castro E.

Fig. 6, lips and buckles of the newborn (Bruhn 1944). Drawn by Castro E.

2. CHARACTERISTICS AND RELATIONSHIPS BETWEEN THE JAWS BETWEEN THE AGES OF 0 AND 5 YEARS.
MONTHS.

A) GENERAL CHARACTERISTICS OF THE JAWS.

In relation to the jaws and orofacial area of the infant, four features of clinical interest stand out during this period:

Maxillary micrognathism: The jaws are small to accommodate the primary teeth, so during the first six months of life there will be an intense three-dimensional growth of them, which will allow the correct eruption and location of the incisors.

❖ **Mandibular retrognathism:** The child is born with the mandible in a retrusive position with respect to the maxilla and there is a distal relationship of the mandibular base with respect to the maxilla.

❖ **Incisal crowding:** An occlusal X-ray shows crowding of the incisor germs in the newborn.

❖ **Intermolar diastemas:** The molars are also vertically overlapping with a scale-like overlap, but there are usually some diastemas between the first and second primary molar in the final θ eruptive phase.

B) RELATIONS BETWEEN THE JAWS.

At this stage of development it is not possible to speak of a true occlusion, as the teeth have not yet erupted, the upper and lower cushions contact in a large part of the dental arches but not in a precise and regular way, so there is a great variety of relations between them, so that they are not a reliable reference.

Some studies claim that an anterior open bite of the pads would be normal. Others claim that there is no relationship between the jaws in the anteroposterior plane, as the mandible is most of the time at rest.

Finally, there are authors who describe the existence of various types of "occlusion" which will influence future occlusion, however, there is no scientific evidence that this is maintained throughout the development and growth of the individual.

One of the most classic classifications is that of Schwarz, which is necessary to mention because it is mentioned by many authors. According to this classification, we could find the following relationships between the dental arches:

I) **SCALON OCLUSION:** Corresponds to the most frequent relationship and according to the orientation of the incisor platform, two types can be distinguished:

FLAT SCALONED OCLUSION: In this case, the incisor platform is horizontal, so that there would be anterior and lateral contact both in centric and during eccentric mandibular movements. The tooth germs are inclined obliquely, which would allow a balanced interlocking in the future θ (Fig. 8).

OBLIC OBLIC OCTION: Here the incisor platform is oblique, so the ridges will only come into contact centrically and not eccentrically. The axes of the tooth germs are in a vertical position θ (Fig. 9).

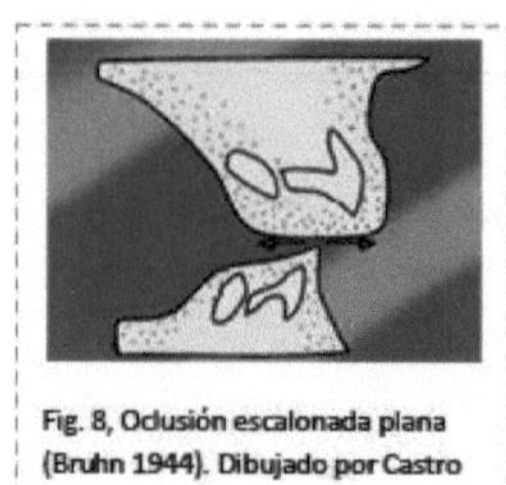

Fig. 8, Oclusión escalonada plana (Bruhn 1944). Dibujado por Castro

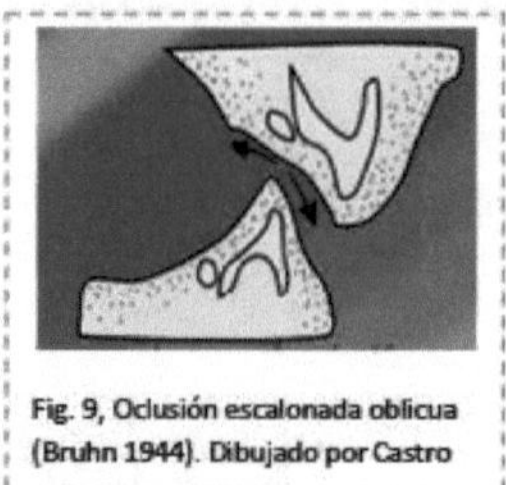

Fig. 9, Oclusión escalonada oblicua (Bruhn 1944). Dibujado por Castro

Fig. 8, Flat stepped occlusion (Bruhn 1944). Drawn by Castro
Fig. 9, Oblique staggered occlusion (Bruhn 1944). Drawn by Castro

II) BOX COVER OCCUSION: In this relationship the incisor platform completely or almost completely covers the lower alveolar process. The germs of the incisors are in a vertical position. This type of relationship, according to its author, could develop into a θ-covered bite in the future (Fig. 10).

III) PROGENIC OCLUSION: In this case, the lower alveolar process is in front of the upper incisor platform, which is due to an incorrect position. of the foetus, which would result in a delay in the development of the upper jaw θ (Fig. 11).

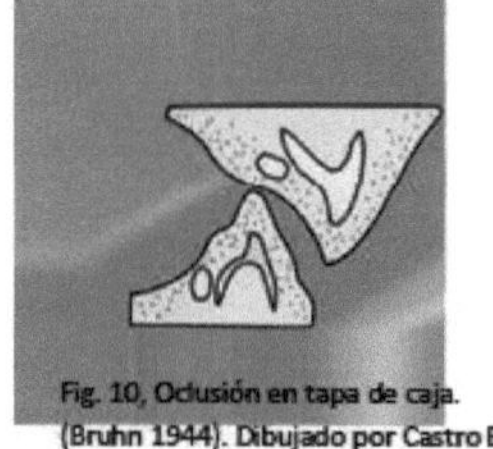

Fig. 10, Oclusión en tapa de caja. (Bruhn 1944). Dibujado por Castro E.

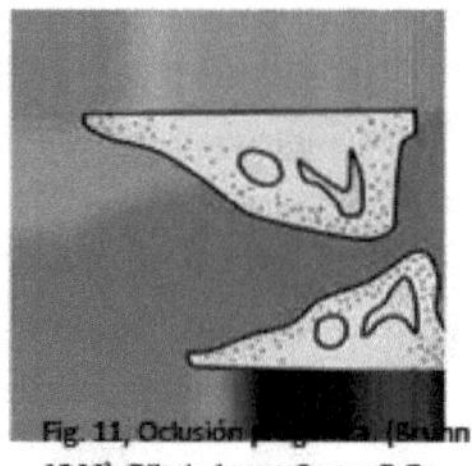

Fig. 11, Oclusión progénica. (Bruhn 1944). Dibujado por Castro E. E.

3. POSITION OF THE TOOTH GERMS INSIDE THE JAWS BETWEEN THE AGES OF 5 MONTHS AND 5 MONTHS.

Between the ages of O and 5 years, the germs of the primary teeth are located in the position that corresponds to them and between them there is a space that will allow their future development. The germs of the upper incisors, according to Korkhaus, can present themselves in different positions, which can vary over time until they reach a location that will allow the correct alignment of the primary teeth in the future. Among the locations described are:

❖ **ALIGNED:** Which would be in the most appropriate position to allow a normal evolution of the position of the teeth in the future.

❖ **APIÑADOS Y ESCALONADOS:** If they remain in this position, they could develop into an inverted bite.

❖ **CLAMPED AND ROTATED:** If they remain in this position, they could evolve to generate frontal compression and dental crowding θ (Fig.12).

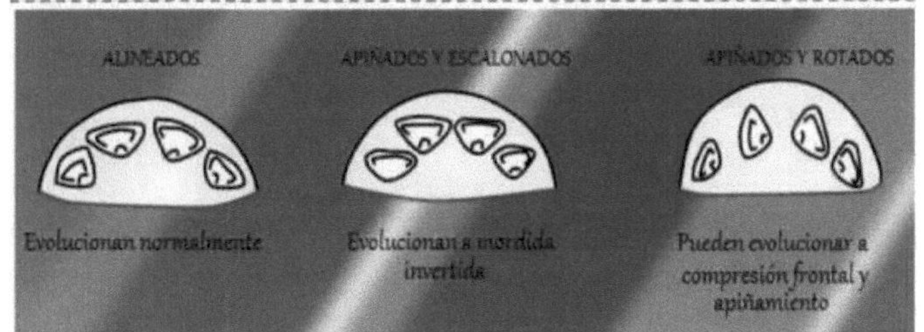

Fig. 12, Position of the dental germs and their possible evolution according to Korkhaus (Leiva 1994). Drawn by Castro E.

LEVEL OF CALCIFICATION OF TEETH AT BIRTH.

At birth the primary teeth and the first permanent molar are calcified as follows (Fig. 13):

A) **Primary central incisors:** crown almost completely calcified.

B) **Primary lateral incisors:** two thirds of the crown calcified.

(c) **Primary canines:** cusp calcified.

D) First primary molar: calcified crown calcification.

E) **Second primary molar:** calcified only at the cusps.

F) **First permanent molar:** apex of mesiovestibular cusp^-

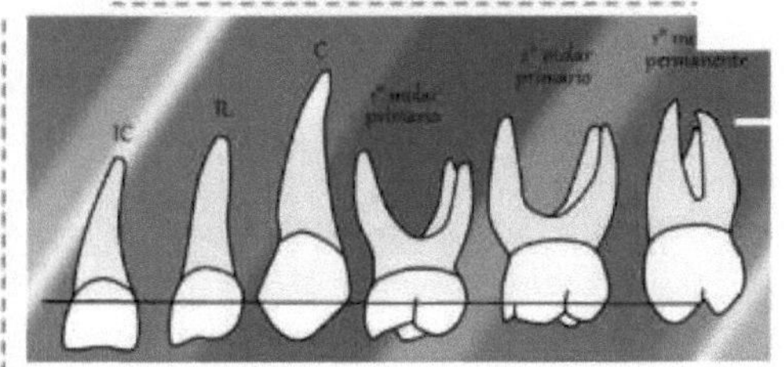

Fig. 13, Level of calcification of the teeth when making (Navarrete 1994). Drawn by Castro E.

13

5. BREASTFEEDING

Breastfeeding is a physiological, complex and neurologically coordinated function that consists of obtaining milk from the mammary gland, this mechanism of muscular action is governed by reflex actions by means of which the child feeds. Breastfeeding takes place in two phases:

❖ **First phase:** There is prehension of the nipple, areola and tight closure of the lips. The lower jaw descends somewhat and a vacuum is formed in the anterior region, the posterior part remaining closed by the soft palate and the posterior part of the tongue (Fig. 14).

❖ **Second phase:** The lower jaw advances from a resting position to place its alveolar ridge in front of the upper jaw. To express the milk, the lower jaw presses on the nipple and squeezes it by rubbing it anteriorly and posteriorly. The tongue takes the form of a spoon, sliding the milk down to the palate (Fig. 15).

Multiple studies have described the benefits of breastfeeding, in the dental field it is mentioned that it allows an adequate growth and development of the oral apparatus, stimulating the musculature favourably through the mechanical work involved in the suction and swallowing that is generated during breastfeeding, which allows the proper mandibular positioning and transverse growth of the jaws, providing a suitable environment for the future development of dental occlusion ^θ·.

Breastfeeding is a stimulus that promotes the advancement of the upper jaw from its distal position relative to the upper jaw to a mesial position. This is the so-called **"first physiological advancement of occlusion"**[7].

It has also been shown that breastfeeding, from birth and for a period of more than 6 months, contributes significantly to the prevention of dental alterations.

- patients who have been bottle-fed from birth or before the age of 6 months have a greater chance of suffering from malocclusions, especially those associated with parafunctional habits.

Another benefit of breastfeeding is reflected in the positive effect it has on the synchronisation of the functions of the oral apparatus. A study in Chile concluded that infants breastfed for more than 9 months were less likely to develop phonetic problems, usually associated with open bites, caused by non-nutritive sucking habits ^θ·

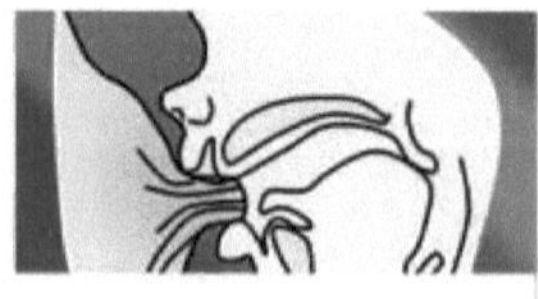

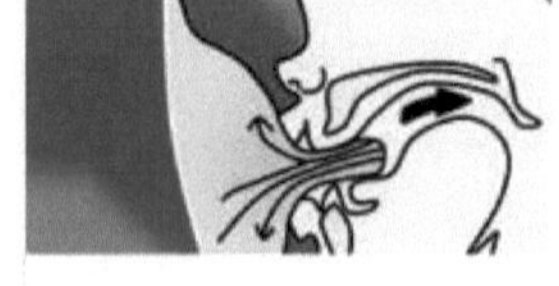

Fig. 14, Primera fase, formación de vacío.
(Bruhn 1944) Dibujado por Castro E.

Fig. 15, Segunda fase, avance mandibular.
(Bruhn 1944), Dibujado por Castro E.

Fig. 14, First phase, vacuum formation (Bruhn 1944) Drawn by Castro E.
Fig. 15, Second phase, mandibular advancement (Bruhn 1944), Drawn by Castro E.

1. What is the role of the Todetessuctional in the baby?
a) Seal the areola during breastfeeding.
b) Allow swallowing during breastfeeding.
c) Allow suction during feeding.
d) Protect the newborn's lips.
2. What is the Robin and Magitot fibrous cord and what is it for?
a) These are structures that cover the alveolar processes and indicate the sites of the developing teeth.
b) These are red-hot protrusions that allow suckling during breastfeeding.
c) They are structures covered with ridges and grooves that contain the germs of the teeth.
d) These are structures located at the level of the corresponding area where incisors and canines will erupt and which facilitate swallowing during suckling.
3. What are the anatomical features of the inferior and superior alveolar ridge respectively?
a) Lower: broad and flattened, upper: narrow and sharp.
b) Lower: narrow and sharp, upper: broad and flattened.
c) Lower: broad and sharp, upper: narrow and flattened.
d) Lower: broad and flattened, upper: broad and flattened.
4. Which anatomical structures of the palate facilitate breastfeeding?
a) Gingival pads.
b) CordonfibrosodeRobinyMagitot.
c) Palatine weatherstripping.
d) Incisive platform.
5. Why is it not possible to speak of occlusion during the 5-month stage, according to the text?
a) Because studies indicate that there is no stable relationship between the maxilla and the mandible.
b) Because there can be multiple possible relationships between Iosmaxillaries.
c) Because at this age not all teeth have erupted yet.
d) Because it has been found that there is a prevalence of open bite in newborns.
6. Which of these characteristics correspond to the "oblique staggered occlusion" according to Schwarz?
a) The incisal platform is oblique, the ridges contact only in centric and the germs are in vertical position.
b) The incisor platform is horizontal, the ridges contact only eccentrically and the germs are in an oblique position.
c) The incisal platform is oblique, the ridges contact in centric and eccentric and the germs are in oblique position.
d) The incisor platform covers almost the entire lower alveolar ridge, the ridges contact only centrically, the germs are in a vertical position.
7. What can be expected to happen in the future with the relationship of the jaws of a

newborn with a progenital relationship, according to the text?

a)   Let it evolve with an open bite.

b)   May develop into anterior inverted bite.

c)   There can be no assurance that this relationship will be sustained over time.

d)   To evolve to Angle Class III.

8.   What could a crowded and staggered incisor placement according to Korkhaus evolve into?

a)   In frontal compression and dental crowding.

b)   In open bite.

c)   In reverse bite.

d)   In crossbite and dental crowding.

9.   What is the level of calcification of teeth at birth?

a)   Primary teeth and first permanent molar almost completely calcified.

b)   Part of calcified primary teeth plus calcified mesiovestibular cusp of first permanent molar.

c)   Part of calcified primary teeth plus calcified mesiovestibular cusp of permanent second molar.

d)   All primary teeth and part of all permanent teeth are calcified.

10. Which of these alternatives is correct about breastfeeding?

a)   It is divided into two phases: in the first phase the jaw is advanced and in the second phase it is hermetically sealed.

b)   It can be replaced by a bottle during the first six months of age without consequences for future growth and development of the oral apparatus.

c)   Contributes to the prevention of dento-buco-maxillo-facial disorders.

d)   May cause phonetic problems in children breastfed for more than 9 months.

SOLUTIONS TO THE SECOND UNIT TEST.

1.   a) Seal the areola during breastfeeding.

2.   b) They are structures located at the level of the corresponding area where incisors and canines will erupt to facilitate swallowing during suckling.

3.   b) Lower: narrow and sharp, upper: broad and flattened.

4.   (c) Palatal weatherstrips.

5.   c) Because not all teeth have erupted at this age.

6.   a) The incisal platform is oblique, the ridges contact only in centric and the germs are in vertical position.

7.   c) There can be no assurance that this relationship will be sustained over time.

8.   (c) In reverse bite.

9.   (b) Part of calcified primary teeth plus calcified mesiovestibular cusp of first permanent molar.

10. c) Contributes to the prevention of dento-buco-maxillofacial disorders.

UNIT III: PRIMARY DENTITION 6 MONTHS TO 2 YEARS OF AGE
AGE.

Objectives
By the end of this unit you will be able to explain:

1) ERUPTION IN PRIMARY DENTITION.

In a simple way, dental eruption corresponds to the moment when the tooth appears in the mouth. Strictly speaking, this term represents a series of phenomena by which the tooth migrates from its place inside the jaws to its position in the oral cavity. This whole process begins with the formation of the tooth germs, however, the axial movement of the teeth is relatively rapid when root development begins. When the length of the root is between half and 2/3 of the final length, the crown approaches the oral cavity and when the tooth pierces the gum, the oral and dental epithelium fuse and cleave exposing the tooth, allowing it to appear in the oral cavity without the gum ulcerating.

In addition to root growth, many theories have been proposed as to the factors responsible for tooth eruption, however, since all these processes occur at the same time, eruption is said to be the result of an interrelationship between all these factors, with root growth and alveolar processes being the essential factors in much of the eruption process.

There are three phases of eruption:

❖ **Pre-eruptive phase:** This corresponds to the stage in which crown calcification is completed, root formation begins and there is intra-alveolar migration towards the oral cavity.

❖ **Pre-functional eruptive phase:** The tooth is present in the mouth without establishing contact with the antagonist.

❖ **Functional eruptive phase:** The tooth establishes occlusion with the antagonist.

2) EMERGENCY DENTAL EMERGENCIES.

This term is used to identify when a tooth cuts or pierces the gum and appears in the oral cavity, but has no more than 3 mm visible (or a quarter of the total size of its crown in incisors and posteriors when the cusps are visible).

3) CHRONOLOGY OF THE ERUPTION OF THE PRIMARY DENTITION.

The eruption of each tooth does not have a precise date, but rather, they are averages of ages. It is more common for the lower teeth to precede the upper teeth; there is variability due to the intervention of various factors, such as race, sex, climate, nutrition, systemic affections and others. The chronology of eruption of the primary teeth is subject to more pronounced genetic influences than for the permanent dentition, and therefore has narrower margins of variability $-.

There are several authors who give different dates for the chronology of the eruption of the primary teeth, we will mention those used by Canut, and also enclosed are the tables of the chronologies of eruption used by Logan and Kronfeld modified by McCall and Schour (Table 1) and by the paediatric dentistry department of the Faculty of Dentistry of the University of Chile (Table 2).

It is worth mentioning that in a study carried out in Chilean children, it was seen that although the eruption sequence was the same as mentioned in the foreign literature, in general there was a delay of 3 months according to the periods mentioned.

The eruption process takes place in three uninterrupted periods:

First group: eruption of lower centrals at 6 months, upper centrals and laterals and finally lower laterals. There is an interval of usually 2 to 3 months between each pair of homologous teeth. Once the incisors have erupted there is a rest period of 4-6 months. At the completion of the eight incisors there is an anterior stop for the mandibular function[®]- During the eruption of the incisor group there is gingival retraction, giving them space for positioning, so that there is no increase in vertical dimension, and the lateral alveolar ridges continue to maintain contact 3' [®] (Fig. 16).

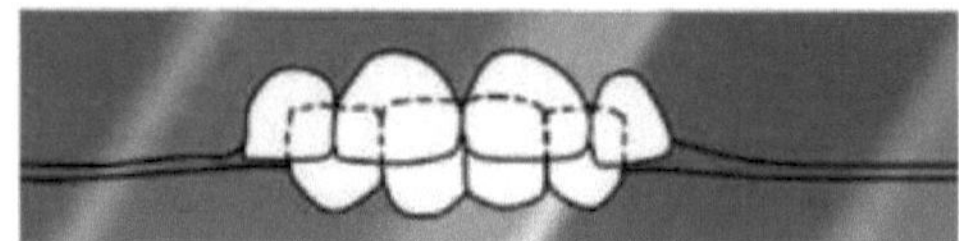

Fig. 16, First group, primary incisors (Reichenbach 1965).
Drawn by Castro E.

Second group: the first primary molars erupt at around 16 months and the canines at around 20 months. The eruption period is 6 months and is followed by a silent period of 4 to 6 months [®]- The eruption of the first primary molar allows the ***FIRST PHYSIOLOGICAL LIFTING OF THE OCCUSION*** to take place (Fig. 17), losing the contact between the alveolar ridges [®]-

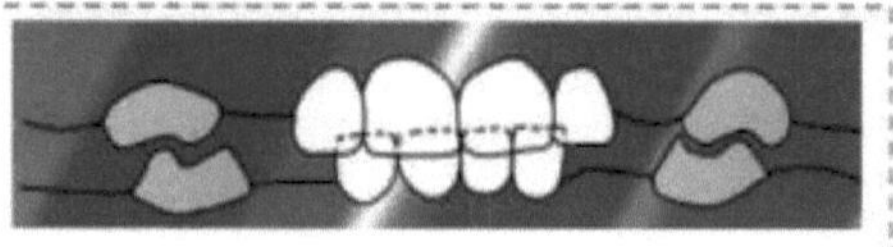

Fig. 17, First physiological raising of the occlusion (Reichenbach 1965). Drawn by Castro E.

Third group: the four second molars erupt, which take about 4 months, and the primary dentition is complete by the age of 2.5 years.

Teeth primary	. ■ ■ home training hard tissue	Amount of enamel	Finished enamel	c · Eruption (months	Root ends da
TABLE 1: Chronology of the development of the primary dentition according to Logan and					
Superiors					
Incisor	14 (13-15)	5/6	1½	8-12	*1*
Incisor	16 (14 2/3-16	2/3	2½	9-13	*2*
Canine	17 (15-18)	1/3	9	16-	3
1st molar	15½(14½-	occlusal	6	13-	2
2° molar	19 (16 -23 ½)	Vertices	11	14-	3
Incisor	14(13-16)	3/5	2½	6-	1
Incisor	16 (14 2/3-16	3/5	3	10-	1
Canine	17 (16-18)	1/3	9	15-	3
1st molar	15 ½	occlusal	5½	14-	2
2° molar	18 (17-19	Vertices	10	23 -	3

TABLE 2: Chronology of eruption in Primary Dentition used by Area of		
Teeth	*Maxilla*	*Jaw*
Central incisor	6-10	5-8
Lateral incisor	8-12	7-10
Canines	16-	
I^{0} Molar	11-	
2 Molar^{o}	20-	

4) GROWTH AND DEVELOPMENT OF DENTAL ARCHES.

The proper development of the dentition depends on the proper growth of the jaws, and the shape and size of the dental arches is determined by several factors, among which are the growth and development of the basal bone of the jaws, the extra- and intra-oral muscular forces, the growth of the alveolar bone that occurs during the eruption of the teeth, and the inclination of the teeth, especially the incisors^-.

The transverse development of both jaws can take place mainly due to the existence of the suture in the medial plane of the maxilla and mandible. However, in the case of the mandible, the synchondrosis of the mandible calcifies at six months of age, so that its transverse growth potential is eliminated early, while the medial suture of the maxilla remains until the development of the dentition and facial growth is complete θ·.

Sagittal growth in the mandible is effected by distai apposition and mesial resorption of the ascending branches of the lower jaw, in the upper jaw the alveolar arch grows downwards and outwards in addition to its transverse growth.

The enlargement of the jaws provides sufficient space for the harmonious emergence of the teeth, creating excess space and diastemas between the erupted anterior teeth $-.

The greatest rate of growth of the dental arches is generated from the age of O months to 3 years, in relation to other ages, since it is during this period that the eruption of the primary teeth takes place. During the period of primary dentition the dental arches acquire a shape that is generally semi-circular^-

5)   CHARACTERISTICS OF THE PRIMARY DENTITION BETWEEN 6 MONTHS AND 2 YEARS OF AGE.

The characteristics of the primary dentition as such will be described in the next unit for age 3 years, with the exception of the overjet and overbite which are different for ages 2 and 3 years, and are mentioned below:

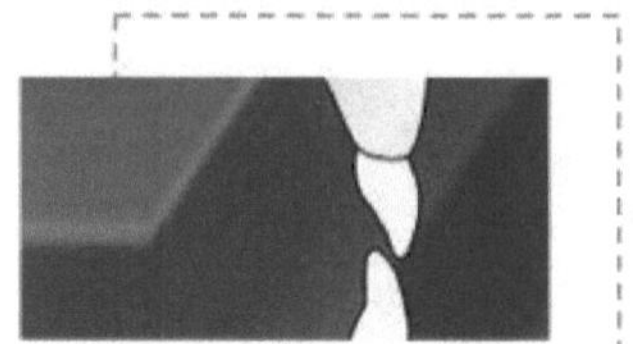

Fig. 18, overjet and overbite at 2 years (Leiva 1994).
Drawn by Castro E.

(A) HIGHLIGHTING, OVERJET OR HORIZONTAL PROJECTION.

The overjet corresponds to the sagittal distance of the vestibular faces of the upper and lower primary incisors from the arches in occlusion Iθ· In a study of Chilean children, the most prevalent overjet was found to be 1 mm 4.

(4) STEP, OVERBITE OR VERTICAL PROJECTION.

The step corresponds to the vertical distance between the edges of the upper and lower primary incisors with the arches in occlusion 15. In a study of Chilean children, the most prevalent step was found to be 1 mm (Fig. 18).

TEST OF THE THIRD UNIT

1.   Which of the following is correct in relation to tooth eruption?

a)   Axial movement of the teeth is relatively rapid when root development begins.

b)   When the root measures ¼ of its final length the crown is close to the oral cavity.

c)   It is used when the tooth cuts or perforates the gum and appears in the mouth.

d)   The pre-eruptive phase is when the tooth is in the mouth without establishing contact with its antagonist.

2.   What is the most important event that occurs when the first primary molars logransu occlude?

a)   Functional eruptive phase is achieved.

b)   An anterior stop for mandibular function is achieved.

c)   The first physiological lifting of the occlusion is achieved.

d)   The first physiological advancement of occlusion is achieved.

3.   What is the order of eruption of the incisor group, according to Canut and Logan and Kronfeld?

a)   I. lower lateral - I. upper lateral - I. upper central - I. lower central.

b)   I. upper lateral - I. lower lateral - I. lower central - I. upper central.

c)   I. lower central - I. upper central - I. upper lateral - I. lower lateral.

d)   I. lateral lower - I. central upper - I. lateral upper - I. central lower.

4.   Between what ages does the highest rate of arch growth take place? dental?

a)   BetweenOmesandS years.

b)   Between 6 months and 3 years.

c)   Between 3 and 6 years.

d)   Between 0 months and 6 years.

5.   What is the most prevalent overjet and overbite at 2 years of age?

a)   Overjet: -1 mm, overbite: 1 mm.

b)   Overjet: lmm, overbite: 1 mm.

c)   Overjet: 1.5 mm, overbite: 2 mm.

d)   Overjet: 0.5 mm, overbite: 1 mm.

SOLUTIONS TO THE THIRD UNIT TEST

1.   a) Axial movement of the teeth is relatively rapid when root development begins.

2.   c) The first physiological occlusal lift is achieved.

3.   (c) lower central I. - upper central I. - upper lateral I. - lower lateral I.

4.   a) Between 0 months and 3 years.

5.   (b) Overjet: lmm, overbite: 1 mm.

UNIT IV: PRIMARY DENTITION AT 3 YEARS OF AGE.

Objectives

By the end of this unit you will be able to explain:

I. The main characteristics of the primary dentition at 3 years of age.

1) CHARACTERISTICS OF THE PRIMARY DENTITIONAT 3 YEARS OF AGE.

The establishment of the primary dentition is generally considered to take place around the age of 3 years, once the roots of the primary second molars have completed their development. From 3 to 4 years of age, the dental arches are relatively stable and changes are slight. The most relevant characteristics of the dentition at 3 years of age will be mentioned below.

A)   SHAPE AND SIZE OF DENTAL ARCHES.

In both jaws the teeth are arranged in a semicircle, which passes from the distal faces of the second primary molars, following the main grooves of the molars, the cusps of the canines and the incisal edges of the anterior teeth. There is also a smaller but not negligible percentage in which the dental arches are elliptical in shape.

In terms of size, the upper dental arch is larger than the lower dental arch, so the teeth of the upper jaw outnumber the teeth of the lower jaw vestibularly.

B)   AXIS OF IMPLANTATION OF THE PRIMARY TEETH IN THE OCCLUSAL PLANE.

The axes of all primary teeth are arranged perpendicular to the occlusal plane 15.

C)   OCCLUSAL PLANE

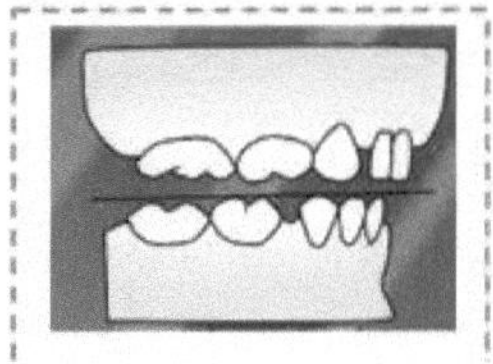

Fig. 19, Occlusal plane at 3 years of age (Navarrete 1993) Drawn by Castro E.

\The occlusal plane in the primary dentition is horizontal (Fig. The edges of incisors, the cusps of primary molars and canines contact in the same plane 15- On the other hand, in the child the morphology of the joint is such that the glenoid cavity is not very marked and the temporal condyle has little relief, so that there is almost no condylar trajectory, therefore the dental arches lack Spee's curve and are rather horizontal Iθ·

D)   INTERPROXIMAL CONTACT RATIO OF THE PRIMARY TEETH.

It is common to find physiological spaces in primary dentition, the most prevalent being the space located mesial to the primary canine in the maxilla and distal to the canine in the mandible, these are also called "primate spaces". Other spaces that can be are called the developmental spaces. These spaces play a fundamental role in the future development of the permanent dentition θ> *14.*

With regard to the reality of our country, a higher frequency of upper primate spaces has been found, in relation to inter-incisor and lower primate 15

E)   OCCLUSAL CONTACT RELATION OF THE PRIMARY TEETH.

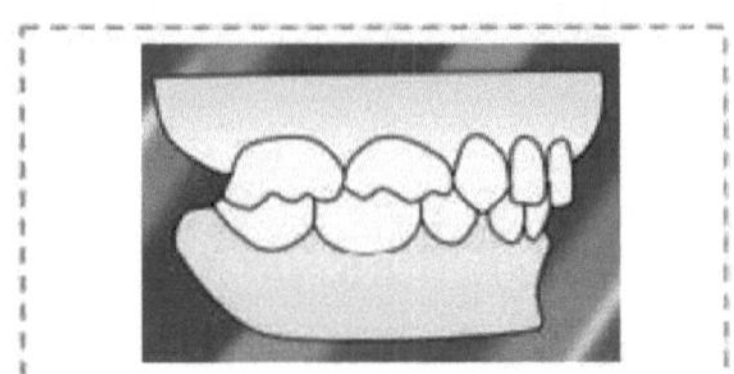

Fig. 20, gear at 3 years of age (Navarrete 1993) Drawn by Castro E.

At this age, a sharp type of meshing is observed, because the primary teeth do not still have wear, so there is a close cusp-fossa θ relationship (Fig. 20).

F)   HIGHLIGHT, OVERJET OR HORIZONTAL PROJECTION.

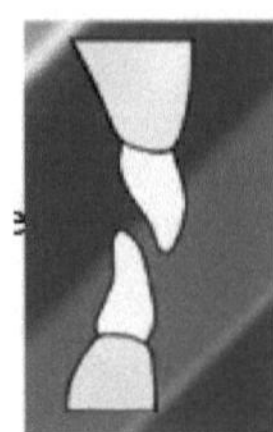

Fig. 21. Overjet and overbite at 3 years of age. Drawn by Castro E.

In studies of Chilean children at this age, the resa
on average 2.6 mm (Fig. 21)

(G) STEP, OVERBITE OR VERTICAL PROJECTION.

Normally the primary incisors are almost perpendicular to the occlusal plane with a slight overbite. Most commonly, the upper primary incisors cover one third of the crown of the lower primary incisors θ. In studies of Chilean children at this age the average step is 2.8 mm 15.

(H) DISTAL RELATIONSHIP OF THE DENTAL ARCHES.

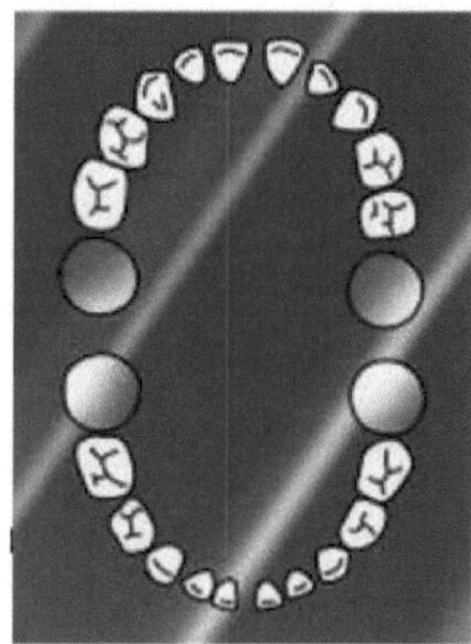

Fig. 22, Campo Molar (Rubio 1989). Drawn by Castro E.

The sagittal distal relationship of the second molars at this age corresponds to the *"postlacteal plane"*, which means that the distal faces of the upper and lower primary second molars are positioned in the same vertical plane θ.

(I) DISTAL LIMIT OF THE SECOND MOLARS

The foreign literature states that at the age of 3 years there is a distal limit to the primary second molars, determined by tuberosity in the maxilla and the branch in the mandible. However,

The reality in Chile shows that there is a space of 9 mm. Distal to the second primary molars 15- This space is called *"molar field" or "retromolar space in the primary dentition"* (Fig. 22), it is formed distal to the second primary molar and will provide space for the future eruption of the first permanent molar Iθ··.

TEST OF THE FOURTH UNIT

1. What is the most prevalent form of the dental arch at 3 years of age?
a) Elliptical
b) Satellite dish
c) Semicircle
d) Circumferential and elliptical.

2. What are "primate spaces"?
a) Physiological spaces located distal to the upper permanent canine and mesial to the lower permanent canine.
b) Physiological spaces located mesial to the upper primary canine and mesial to the lower primary canine.
c) Physiological spaces located mesial to the upper permanent canine and distai lower permanent canine.
d) Physiological spaces located mesial to the upper primary canine and distal to the lower primary canine.

3. What is the occlusal plane like at 3 years of age?
a) It has curvatures, such as Wilson and Spee.
b) It is horizontal.

c)   It has aSpee curvature.

d)   It has a postlacteal plane.

4.   What is the occlusal contact relationship like at 3 years of age?

a)   There is physiological wear and tear so the gear is little stressed.

b)   It has a sharp gearing due to the presence of physiological spaces.

c)   It has an accentuated gearing due to the fact that physiological wear and tear is not yet present.

d)   It is spaced by the presence of primate spaces.

5.   What does the concept of "Campo Molar" refer to?

a)   This refers to the fact that the distal sides of the primary second molars are positioned in the same plane.

b)   Refers to the area that will be formed to accommodate the first permanent molar when it erupts.

c)   Refers to the distal face of the lower primary second molar being mesial to the face of the upper primary second molar.

d)   This refers to the fact that the primary second molars do not end directly with the tuberosity and the mandibular ramus.

SOLUTIONS TO THE FOURTH UNIT TEST.

1.   (c) Semicircle

2.   d) Physiological spaces located mesial to the upper primary canine and distal to the lower primary canine.

3.   b) It is horizontal.

4.   c) It has an accentuated gearing due to the fact that physiological wear and tear is not yet present.

5.   b) Refers to the area to be formed for the first permanent molar to be located when it erupts.

V UNIT: PRIMARY DENTITION AT 5 YEARS OF AGE.

Objectives

By the end of this unit you will be able to explain:

I. The main characteristics of the primary dentition at 5 years of age.

1) CHARACTERISTICS OF THE PRIMARY DENTITION AT 5 YEARS OF AGE.

A)   SHAPE AND SIZE OF DENTAL ARCHES.

The dental arches continue to maintain their semicircular shape, other shapes such as parabolic and elliptical are also less prevalent.

From 5 to 6 years of age the dental arch begins to change due to the eruptive force of the first permanent molar.

B)   AXIS OF IMPLANTATION OF THE PRIMARY TEETH IN THE OCCLUSAL PLANE.

The axes of the primary teeth maintain their arrangement perpendicular to the occlusal plane. Some authors point out that the incisors are vestibularised due to the pressure of the permanent successors during growth.

C)   OCCLUSAL PLANE

It remains horizontal, as the primary teeth remain in the same arrangement, as does the temporomandibular joint.

D) INTERPROXIMAL CONTACT RATIO OF PRIMARY TEETH.

Physiological spaces in the primary dentition continue to be very frequent, and are a fundamental factor for the future eruption and positioning of the permanent incisors. However, it has been shown that this is not an essential factor, as there are cases in which, despite the absence of physiological spaces, the permanent teeth can align without crowding.

(I) OCCLUSAL CONTACT RATIO OF THE PRIMARY TEETH.

By the age of 5 years the primary dentition has undergone wear of the occlusal surfaces of the teeth due to normal masticatory function, so that there will be little pronounced engagement. This wear will allow a proper distal relationship of the primary second molars to develop, contribute a favourable step and protrusion and facilitate mandibular advancement, which is known as the ***"Second Mandibular Advancement"***[16] ·

(F) HIGHLIGHTING, OVERJET 0 HORIZONTAL PROJECTION.

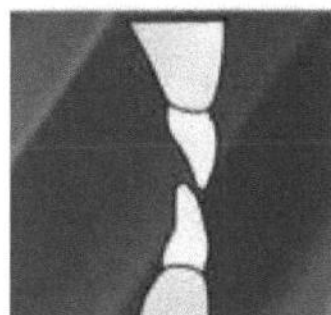

Fig. 23, overjet and overbite at 5 years of age (Rubio 1989) Drawn by Castro E.

The physiological wear and tear characteristic of this age will allow the mesial advancement of the mandible to be generated, which in turn will determine that the overjet or protrusion decreases to 1 mm.

(G) STEP, OVERBITE OR VERTICAL PROJECTION.

Due to the physiological wear and tear and loss of gearing of the primary teeth the overbite decreases to 1 mm (Fig. 23).

(H) DISTAL RELATIONSHIP OF PRIMARY SECOND MOLARS.

In order to classify the occlusion in the primary dentition, the terminal plane is used as a reference, which corresponds to the mesiodistal relationship between the distal surfaces of the upper and lower primary second molars when the teeth are in centric contact.

a) **Level, vertical plane or postlacteal plane:** The relationship where the distal faces of the second molars are in the same vertical plane (Fig. 24).

b) **Mesial step:** the distal surface of the lower molars is more mesial than the upper (Fig. 25).

c) **Distal step:** The distal surface of the lower molars is more distal than the upper θ (Fig. 26).

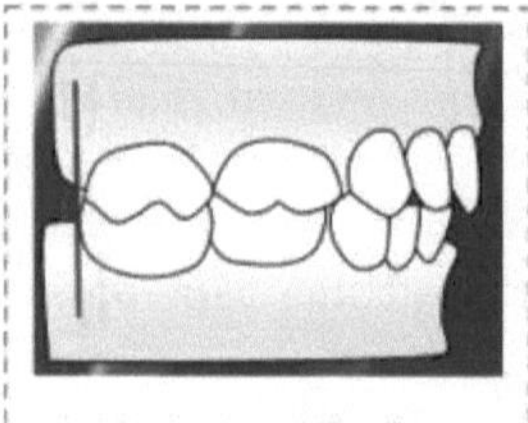

Fig. 24, Plano postlácteo. (Torres 2009). Dibujado por Castro E.

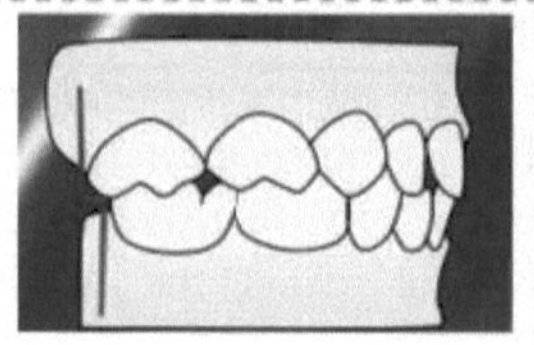

Fig. 25, Escalón mesial. (Torres 2009). Dibujado por Castro E.

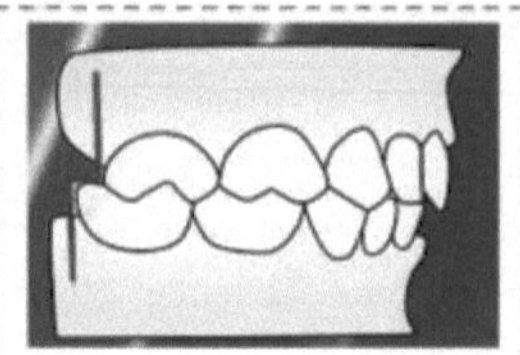

Fig. 26, Escalón distal. (Torres 2009). Dibujado por Castro E.

Fig. 24, Postlacteal plan (Torres 2009). Drawn by Castro E.

Fig. 25, Mesial step (Torres 2009). Drawn by Castro E. Fig. 26, Distai step (Torres 2009). Drawn by Castro E.

(A) DISTAL LIMIT OF THE PRIMARY SECOND MOLARS.

Molar field still present

2) PHYSIOLOGICAL ROOT RESORPTION IN THE PRIMARY DENTITION.

The physiological resorption of primary teeth is an intermittent process that is initiated and stimulated by the eruption of germs from the permanent teeth.

During this process, periods of active resorption, carried out by odontoclasts, alternate with periods of rest, in which repair processes take place to restore the periodontal function of the resorbed area, during which cement is deposited on the root surface.

EST OF THE FIFTH UNIT

1. Why does the second physiological advancement of occlusion occur?

a) Due to physiological wear and tear caused by normal feeding, which allows a displacement of the jaw.

b) Due to the eruptive force of the first permanent molar.

c) Due to mandibular advancement as a result of breastfeeding.

d) Due to the existence of a mesial step relationship between the primary second molars.

2. What are the three relationships we can find between distal faces

of primary second molars at 5 years of age?

a) Postlacteal plane - mesial step - vertical plane.

b) Vertical plane - mesial step - distai step.

c) Mesial step - straight plane - vertical plane.

d) Postlacteal step - mesial plane - distai plane.

3. What is the average overjet and overbite at 5 years of age?

a) Overjet: 2.7, overbite: 2.8

b) Overjet: 2,6 overbite: 2,8

c) Overjet: 2,5 overbite: 2,8

d) Overjet: 1, overbite: 1

4. What are the characteristics of the distal limit of the primary dentition at 5 years of age?

a) Presence of molar field or retromolar space in primary dentition.

b) Presence of postlacteal plane.

c) Presence of physiological spaces for the future eruption of the first permanent molar.

d) Presence of weakly accentuated gearing.

5. What is correct about physiological root resorption in the primary dentition?

a) It is a process of constant active resorption carried out by odontoblasts.

b)   During this process there is no repair to re-establish periodontal function.

c)   It is an intermittent process stimulated by the eruption of germs from the permanent teeth.

d)   It starts when the permanent tooth has a fully formed root.

SOLUTIONS TO THE FIFTH UNIT TEST

1.   a) Due to physiological wear and tear caused by normal feeding which allows a displacement of the jaw.

2.   b) Vertical plane - mesial step - distai step.

3.   (d) Overjet: 1, overbite: 1

4.   a) Presence of molar field or retromolar space in primary dentition.

5.   c) It is an intermittent process stimulated by the eruption of permanent tooth germs.

REFERENCES

1. Sadler T. Langman: Medical Embryology. II⁰ Edition. Barcelona: Wolters Kluwerhealth;2010.P. 265-289.

2. Castillo R., Perona G., Kanashiro C., Perea M., Silva F. Pediatric Stomatology. I⁰ Edition. Madrid: Ripano S.A; 2011. P. 15-21.

3. Reichenbach E., Brückl H. Orthopaedicomaxillary clinic and therapy. 15th edition. Argentina: Editorial Mundi S.A. 1965. P. 12 -26.

4. Leiva N., Cauvi D., Espinoza, A. Characteristics of the primary dentition in children between 6 and 24 months of age. [Thesis for the degree of Surgeon - Dentist]. Santiago: University of Chile, Faculty of Dentistry, Dentomaxillary Orthopaedics. 1994. P. 13 - 17, 35 - 36.

5. Montenegro A., Mery A. and AGUIRRE, A. Histology and embryology of the stomatognathic system. Santiago. Department of Experimental Morphology, Faculty of Medicine, University of Chile. 1983. P. 192,115-116.

6. CanutJ. Clinical Orthodontics. 2° Edition. Barcelona: Elsevier Masson. 2000. P. 43-47.

7. Benitez L., Calvo L., Quiros O., Maza P., Jurisic A., Alcedo C. et al. Study of breastfeeding as a determinant factor in the prevention of dentomaxillofacial anomalies. Latin American Journal of Orthodontics and Paediatric Dentistry. [internet]. 2009. [cited 2015 September 22]. p.

6 - 17. Available from:
https://www.ortodoncia.ws/publicaciones/2009/art20.asp

8. Buhn C., Hofrath H., Korkhaus G. Orthodontics. 2° edition. Barcelona; Editorial Labor. 1944. P. 74-109.

9. Torres M. Development of the dentition. The primary dentition. Latin American Journal of Orthodontics and Paediatric Dentistry. [Internet]. 2009. [cited 2015 Sep 22]. p. 1 - 23. Available from: https://www.ortodoncia.ws/publicaciones/2009/art23.asp

10. Rondon R., Zambrano G., Guerra M. Relationship of breastfeeding and Dento-Buco-Maxillo-Facial development: A review of the Latin American literature. Latin American Journal of Orthodontics and Paediatric Dentistry. [Internet]. 2012. [cited 2015 Sep 22]. P. 2-23. Available from: https://www.ortodoncia.ws/publicaciones/2012/art20.asp

11. Boj J., Catalá M., García-Ballesta C., Mendoza A., Planells P. Odontopediatria, la evolución del niño al adulto joven. I⁰ Edicion. Madrid: RipanoS.A. 2011. P. 76-81.

12. Romero M., Chávez E., Barrero J., Prevalence and sequence of eruption in the lower jaw in selected patients of the U.G.M.A 2006 interceptive orthodontic diploma course. Latin American Journal of Orthodontics and Paediatric Dentistry. [Internet]. 2008. [cited 2015 Sep 22]. P. 2-3. Available from:
https://www.ortodoncia.ws/publicaciones/2008/artl0.asp

13. Pinto M. Anatomía dentaria evolución de la dentición. Practical Guide. University of Chile, Faculty of Dentistry, Subject of Paediatric Dentistry. 2013.

14. Nakata M., Wei S. Guía Oclusal en Odontopediatria. I⁰ Edición, Venezuela; Actualidades medico odontologicas S.A. 1992. P.7 -14.

15. Navarrete M., Cauvi D., Espinoza, A. Characteristics of the Normal Temporal Dentition at three years of age. [Thesis for the degree of Surgeon - Dentist]. Santiago: University of Chile,

Faculty of Dentistry, Dentomaxillary Orthopaedics. 1993. P. 17 - 23, 53 -58.

16. Rubio L., Cauvi D., Espinosa A. Characteristics of the Temporary Dentition in Normality, at the age of 5 years. Thesis for the degree of Surgeon - [Tesis para optar al título de Cirujano Dentist]. Santiago: University of Chile, Faculty of Dentistry,

Subject: Dentomaxillary Orthopaedics. 1989. P.3- 14, 38 -56.

CHAPTER 2

MIXED DENTITION FIRST PHASE
I UNIT: IMPORTANT CONCEPTS.

Objectives

By the end of this unit you will be able to explain:

1. *The concepts of tooth eruption in the permanent dentition* and *mixed dentition first phase.*

1) ERUPTION IN THE PERMANENT DENTITION.

The concept of eruption for the permanent dentition is the same as for the primary dentition, however, during the eruption of permanent teeth there is greater variability, due to hormonal factors and gender difference. It is classically accepted that the first permanent tooth to erupt is the first permanent molar, then incisors, and finally the lateral sectors are replaced. In general, the eruption of permanent teeth will be completed as follows:

❖ The permanent anterior teeth will develop lingually from the primary teeth and close to their apex, their migration will start when root formation begins.

In their path, the permanent incisors meet the root of the primary teeth, which they reabsorb, to later erupt through the labial of these, generally. It is common for the crowns of the primary incisors to remain in the mouth when the permanent teeth have erupted and if they have already exfoliated, the permanent teeth will reopen the gum. Due to their eruption path, permanent teeth are usually more buccally inclined than their primary predecessors.

❖ Premolars will also develop lingually from the dental lamina of the primary molars and emerge between their roots, erupted in a slightly mesial position and their crown will be exposed to the buccal environment after the exfoliation of the primary molars.

❖ The permanent molars originate from a distal proliferation of the dental lamina of the second primary molars and emerge with a distal inclination K

2) MIXED DENTITION FIRST PHASE.

Mixed dentition is the stage of dentition in which *both primary and permanent* teeth are present in the oral cavity.

The mixed dentition is divided into mixed dentition first stage and mixed dentition second stage.

The first stage of mixed dentition, which will be discussed in this chapter, is the stage that goes from approximately *5.5 to 9 years* of age and includes the eruption of the *first permanent molars and incisors.*

TEST OF THE FIRST UNIT

1. Why is there greater variability in the eruption of the permanent dentition than in the primary dentition?
a) Because it is mostly influenced by genetic factors.
b) Because their eruption tends to be more difficult.
c) The presence of racial and socio-economic factors.
d) Due to the presence of hormonal factors and sex differences.
2. What is the first permanent tooth to erupt, according to the text?
a) Lower central incisor.
b) Lower lateral incisor.

30

c) Primermolarpermanent.

d) Upper central incisor.

3. Which of the following alternatives is correct in relation to the rash
of previous permanent teeth?

a) During eruption, they follow the same path as primary teeth as they are resorbed.

b) They usually erupt labially from the primary teeth.

c) They erupt slightly mesial to the primary teeth.

d) They erupt slightly different from the primary teeth.

4. What is the approximate age range for the first stage of mixed dentition?

a) From 5.5 to 9 years of age.

b) From 4 to 9 years of age.

c) From 5.5 to 12 years of age.

d) From 7 to 10 years of age.

5. What teeth can we find in the mouth during the first stage of mixed dentition?

a) Permanent incisors and first molars.

b) Primary teeth, incisors and first permanent molars.

c) Permanent incisors and second molars.

d) Primary incisors and permanent first molars.

SOLUTIONS TO THE FIRST UNIT TEST

1. d) Due to the presence of hormonal factors and sex difference.

2. c) First permanent molar.

3. b) Generally erupt labially from the primary teeth.

4. a) From 5.5 to 9 years of age.

5. b) Primary teeth, incisors and first permanent molars.

UNIT II: EVOLUTION OF THE FIRST PERMANENT MOLAR

> **Objectives**
>
> *By the end of this unit you will be able to explain:*
>
> I. *The importance of the permanent first molar in occlusion.*
>
> II. *The development* and *eruption of the first permanent molar.*
>
> III. *The possible occlusal relationships that can be acquired from the permanent first molar.*

1) IMPORTANCE OF THE FIRST PERMANENT MOLAR

The first permanent molars are the most important teeth, as they are the first permanent teeth to appear in the mouth, they also play a fundamental role in the development and functionality of the permanent dentition, among which we can mention:

❖ They account for 50% of masticatory efficiency.

❖ They serve as a guide for eruption and positioning of the molar group.

❖ They produce the second physiological raising of the occlusion 3'4,5.

❖ It is considered "The key to occlusion" 5.

The loss of this tooth generates alterations in the dental balance, producing changes in the axes of the rest of the teeth, traumatic occlusion and problems at the temporomandibular joint level^-.

2) DEVELOPMENT AND ERUPTION OF THE FIRST PERMANENT MOLAR.

The organogenesis of the first permanent molar begins around $4°$ month of intrauterine life, from an extension of the dental lamina. At birth, its mesiovestibular cusp is already calcified and its enamel is fully formed between 2.5 and 3 years of age. Its root formation will be completed between 9 and 10 years of age θ.

The germ of the upper first permanent molar develops in the tuberosity of the maxilla and its occlusal surface is oriented downwards and backwards, while the germ of the lower first permanent molar is positioned in the angle of the mandible and its occlusal surface is oriented upwards and forwards, which determines a difference in the eruption pattern of both. When the first permanent molar erupts it contacts the distal surface of the second primary molar, however this location is unstable until the intercuspid relationship between the upper and lower first permanent molars is achieved.

As mentioned above, the space for the eruption of the first permanent molar is produced by a posterior growth distal to the dental arches, called the ***molar field, which*** is formed by apposition in the area of the tuberosity and resorption of the anterior part of the ramus, compensated by apposition in its posterior part 5> (Fig. 27).

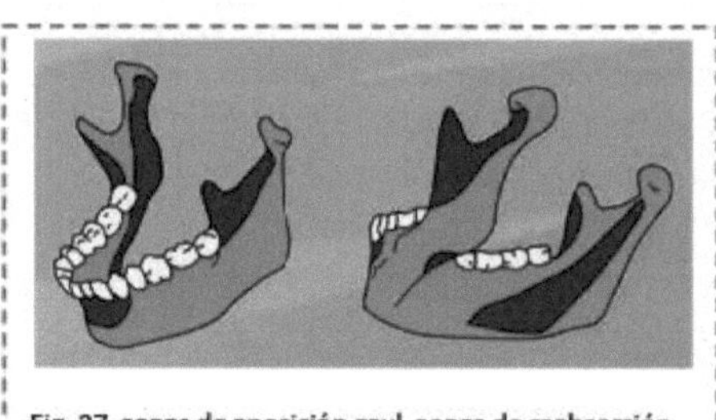

Fig. 27, zonas de aposición azul, zonas de reabsorción verde. (Moyers 1992). Dibujado por Castro E.

Fig. 27, blue apposition zones, green resorption zones (Moyers 1992). Drawn by Castro E.

n terms of eruption chronology,

There are differences between the various authors, due to the criteria used in the measurements and the differences between the populations studied 5.

According to the ages proposed by Logan and Kronfeld as modified by McCall and Shour, both the upper and lower first permanent molars erupt between the ages of 6 and 7 years 1, whereas according to the chronology used by

the area of Dentistry of the University of Chile, erupt between 5.5 and 7 years of age^.

Teeth	Home hard tissue formation	Quantity of enamel at birth	Finished enamel	Eruption	Finished root
TABLE 2: Chronology of the development of the Permanent Dentition according to Logan and Kronfeld, slightly modified by McCall and Schour ĸ					
I° MS	Birth	Sometimes a	2½-3	6-7 years	9-10 years
I° MI	Birth	Sometimes a	2½-3	6-7 years	9-10 years

TABLE4: Eruption chronology in permanent dentition used by		
Teeth **Permanent**	**Maxilla (years)**	**Mandible (years)**
I⁰ Molar		5.5 -

Studies carried out by professors of the Faculty of Dentistry of the University of Chile have concluded that the dates of eruption of the first permanent molar are divided both by dental arches and by sex. For the latter parameter, the following values were determined on average:

❖ Women: 5.6 to 6 years
❖ Males: 6.1 to 6.5 years[3] .

In general, the mandibular molars erupt before the upper molars, while no significant differences are observed in the hemiarchs. The fact that it occurs first in females could be explained by the greater sexual and skeletal development that they present with respect to males at this stage of growth[3] .

Once the first permanent molars have erupted and have reached the occlusal plane, the **Second Physiological Lift of laOclusion** is generated[3] ,5.

3) OCCLUSAL RELATIONSHIPS OF THE FIRST PERMANENT MOLAR.

The way the first permanent molars will occlude can be predicted from the relationship between the distal surfaces of the second primary molars. The relationship between the types of planes and the early occlusion of the first molars can be Λ

A) VERTICAL STRAIGHT PLANE OR POSTLATIAL PLANE: The terminal relationship of the second primary molars is vertical (Fig. 27), their surfaces will guide the first permanent molars to an unstable position which could lead to an initial *cuspid to cuspid* relationship that will later be transformed into a neutroclusion relationship, i.e. *cuspid to fossa.* Among the theories explaining how this would originate are: θ>.

I)   Closure of the primate spaces: The presence of physiological spaces located between lateral incisors and primary canines in the maxilla (Fig. 28), and between canines and primary first molars in the mandible, would allow the passage from a *straight terminal plane* to a *mesial step,* necessary to allow neutroclusion of the first permanent molars θ>.

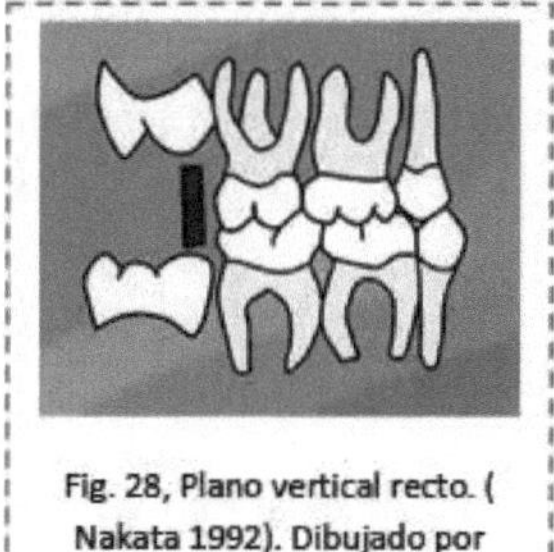

Fig. 28, Plano vertical recto. (Nakata 1992). Dibujado por Castro E.

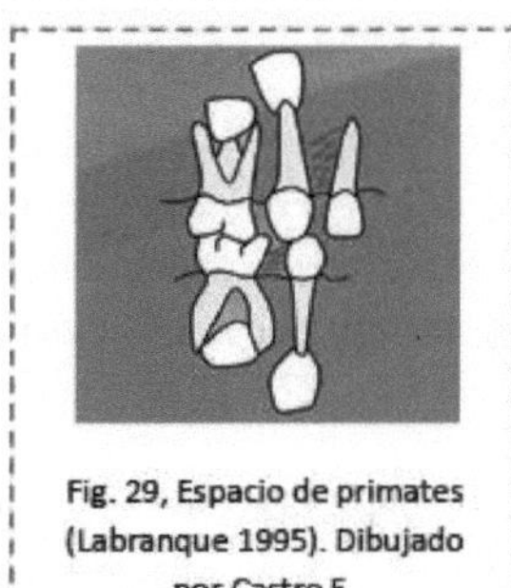

Fig. 29, Espacio de primates (Labranque 1995). Dibujado por Castro E.

II)   Mesial advancement of the mandible: The physiological wear of the incisal edges of the primary teeth would determine the loss of the meshing between acute cusps and fossae or sulci, which would produce a *mesial advancement of the mandible* (Fig. 30), allowing the neutroclusion of the first permanent molars.

III) Late mesial shift: There is a mesial shift of the first permanent molars to close the spaces generated by a larger mesiodistal diameter of the space occupied by primary canines and molars in relation to the diameter occupied by permanent canines and premolars θ> (Fig. 31).

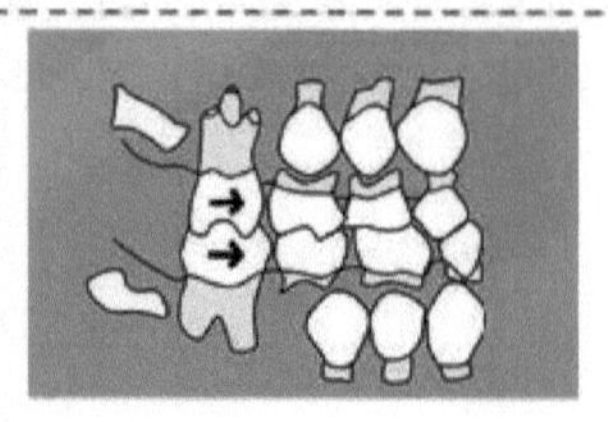

Fig. 30, Avance mesial de la mandíbula. (Labranque 1995). Dibujado por Castro E.

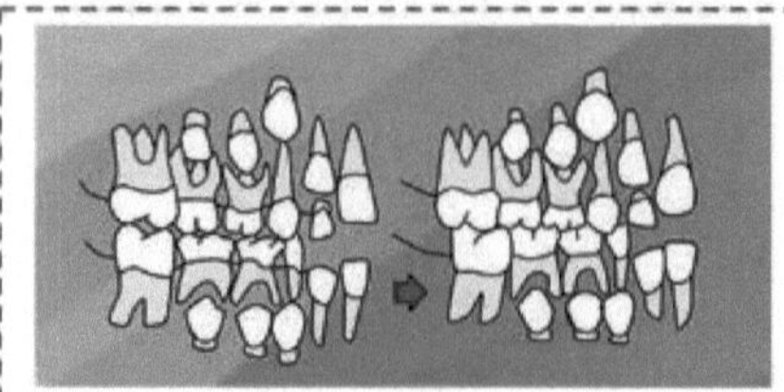

Fig. 31, Desplazamiento mesial tardío. (Labranque 1995). Dibujado por Castro E.

IV) Combination of two or more processes: Two or more of the above mentioned processes occur 5.

V) Anatomical shape of the teeth: There are *inclined planes* that cause the mesiopalatal cusp of the upper first permanent molar to be directed more and more inwards into the fossa of the lower first permanent molar during eruption, allowing neutroclusion to be achieved (Fig. 32).

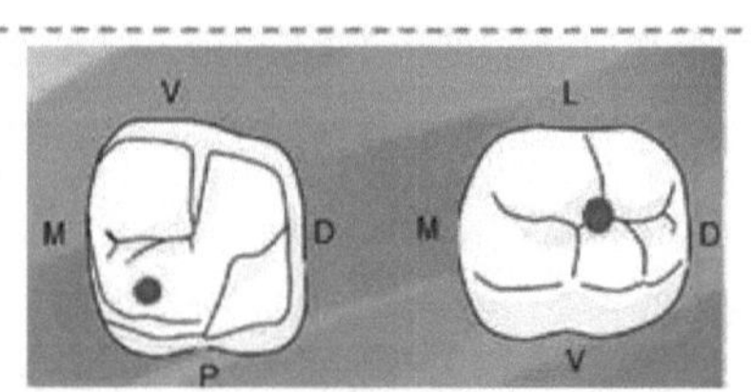

Fig. 32, Forma anatómica de las piezas dentarias. (Labraque 1995). Dibujado por Castro E.

Fig. 32, Anatomical shape of the teeth (Labraque 1995). Drawn by Castro E.

B) MESIAL SCALO: This is the most frequently occurring type of occlusal relationship. In this case, the *distal surface of the lower primary second molar is mesial to the distal surface of the upper primary second molar* (Fig. 33).

The mesial step ensures correct intercuspidation of the permanent molar, as it will allow neutroclusion of the first permanent molars from the beginning.

The mesial step is due to the fact that the upper incisors move labially between the ages of four and six years producing a lengthening of the dental arch, which would allow the lower jaw to adopt a more mesial position, which is further facilitated when there is greater abrasion of the occlusal surfaces of the primary teeth. This process is called **Second Physiological Advancement of Occlusion**[5].

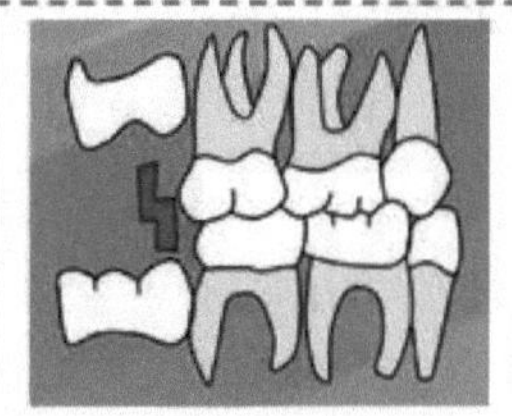

Fig. 33, Escalón mesial y
Neutroclusión. (Labranque 1995).
Dibujado por Castro E.

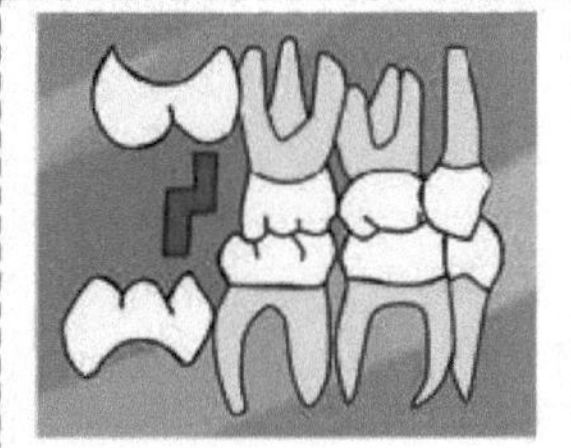

Fig. 34, Escalón distal y
distoclusión. (Labranque 1995).
Dibujado por Castro E.

Fig. 33, Mesial step and Neutroclusion (Labranque 1995). Drawn by Castro E.
Fig. 34, Distai step and distoclusion (Labranque 1995). Drawn by Castro E.

C) DISTAL STAGE: In this case the *distal surface of the second lower primary molar is distal to the distal surface of the upper primary molar.* This relationship between the primary molars is not considered normal, as it could lead to distoclusion of the first permanent molars (Fig.34).

TEST OF THE SECOND UNIT

1. Why does the "Second physiological raising of the occlusion" occur?
a) Eruption of the first permanent molar.
b) For the occlusion between the first four permanent molars.
c) For the masticatory efficiency of the first permanent molar.
d) The involvement of the first permanent molar as the "key to occlusion".

2. When does organogenesis of the first permanent molar begin?
a) During the 4th° month of life after birth.
b) During the 6° month of intrauterine life.
c) During the 4th⁰ week of intrauterine life.
d) During the 4th° month of intrauterine life.

3. Between what ages does the first permanent molar erupt according to the chronology used by Logan and Kronfeld?
a) Between 6 and 7 years.
b) Between 4 and 7 years old.
c) Between 6 and 8 years old.
d) Between 5 and 9 years old.

4. What is correct about the eruption of the first permanent molar?
a) There are no gender differences.
b) No significant differences were found according to hemiarchs.
c) The mandibular first molar usually erupts after the upper first molar.
d) It usually erupts first in males rather than females.

5. Why does "Late Mesial Displacement" occur?
a) The presence of physiological spaces mesial to the upper primary canine and distal to the lower primary canine.
b) Due to physiological wear of the primary teeth.

c) Due to the inclined planes on the cusps of the permanent first molars.

d) Due to the larger mesiodistal diameter of primary canines and molars in relation to permanent canines and premolars.

6. Which of these relationships between the distal faces of the primary second molars ensures neutroclusion of the permanent first molars from the beginning?

a) Mesial Step.

b) Distai Step.

c) Postlacteal plane.

d) Mesial advancement of the mandible.

7. Which of these relationships between the distal faces of the primary second molars could lead to a distoclusion between the permanent first molars?

a) Mesial Step.

b) Postlacteal plane.

c) Planovertical.

d) Distai Step.

SOLUTIONS TO THE SECOND UNIT TEST

1. b) By the occlusion between the first four permanent first molars.

2. d) During the 4th° month of intrauterine life.

3. (a) Between 6 and 7 years.

4. b) No significant differences were found according to hemiarchs.

5. d) Due to the larger mesiodistal diameter of primary canines and molars in relation to permanent canines and premolars.

6. a) Mesial Step.

7. d) Distai step.

III UNIT: EVOLUTION OF THE PERMANENT INCISORS

Objectives

By the end of this unit you will be able to explain:

I.   The development and eruption of permanent incisors.

II.   The replacement of the primary incisor group by the permanent incisor group and what factors allow this to happen.

III.   The characteristics of the incisor group during the first stage mixed dentition.

IV.   The characteristics of the protrusion and step in permanent incisors.

TABLE 5: Chronology of the development of the permanent dentition according to					
Teeth	Home hard tissue formation	Γ,A d Quantity of enamel at birth	Finished enamel	c ■■ Eruption	Finished root
Incisor	3-4	-	4-5	7-8 years	10 years
Incisor	10-12	-	4-5	8-9	11 years
Incisor	3-4	-	4-5	6-7	9 years
Incisor	3-4	-	4-5	7-8	10 years
TABLE 6: Eruption Chronology in Permanent Dentition used by					
Teeth Permanent		Maxilla (years)		Mandible (years)	

| Central incisor | 7-8 | 6-7 |
| Lateral incisor | 8-9 | 7-8 |

2) CHANGE OF THE INCISORS.

The change of the primary incisors starts with the lower central incisor. The sum of the mesiodistal width of the four permanent incisors is greater than that of the four primary incisors, which is approximately 7 mm in the upper jaw and approximately 5 mm in the lower jaw, which is why certain changes in the dental arch must occur for the correct alignment of the permanent incisors.

During the change of space in the anterior region, the total space in the arch becomes deficient, so there is crowding. The position of the canines and premolars depends on how the permanent incisors are positioned.

There are four Regulatory factors that control the placement of the four permanent incisors
Λ

A)   INTERDENTAL SPACE IN THE REGION OF THE PRIMARY INCISORS.

Physiological spaces are important factors that will facilitate the accommodation in the arch of the relatively large permanent incisors in relation to the primary incisors, if there is no space in the primary dentition, the permanent incisors tend to overcrowd, so the presence or absence of primary spaces will affect the accommodation of the incisors in an important way. 7

B) INCREASE IN INTERCANINE DIAMETER.

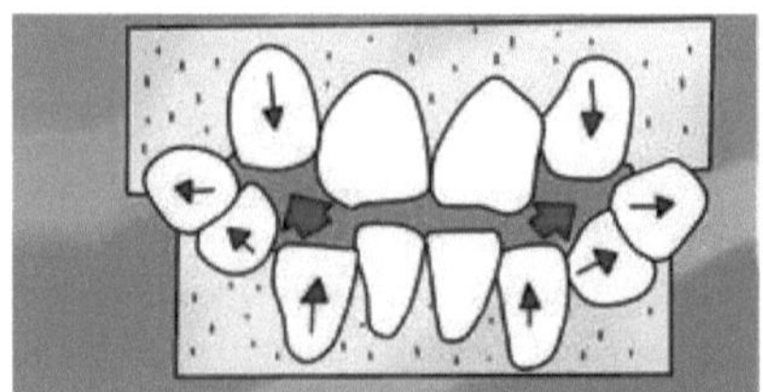

Fig. 35, Increased intercanine diameter (Canut 2000). Drawn by Castro E.

During the period of incisor eruption, an increase in the intercanine width (transverse growth between the canines) can be observed at the time of eruption of the upper central and lower lateral incisors (Fig. 35). When the incisors complete their eruption, the intercanine width increases by approximately 3 mm in each jaw. In the upper jaw the intercanine width increases by a further 1.5 mm when the canines erupt ∧

C) ANTERIOR DENTAL ARCH AUGMENTATION.

There is an increase in the dental arch in an anterior-posterior direction that will allow space for the permanent incisors, which are larger than the primary incisors. The permanent incisors must erupt more labially to achieve the additional space needed (Fig. 36), they move 2 to 3 mm in relation to the primary incisors. In the lower jaw, the permanent incisors are occasionally located lingually to the primary incisors, immediately after erupting ∧

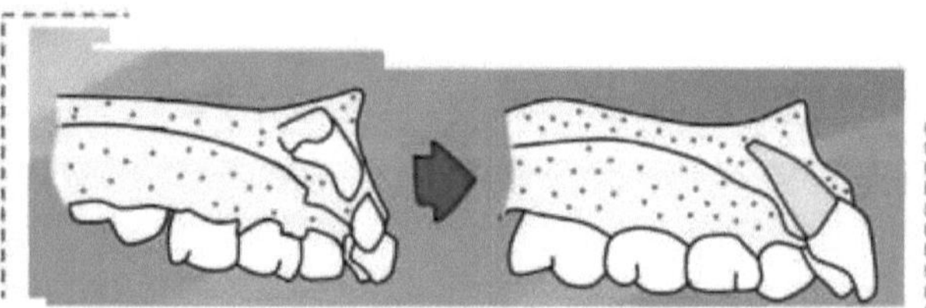

Fig. 36, More vestibular location of the permanent incisors (Canut2000). Drawn by Castro E.

D) CHANGE IN THE AXIS OF THE PERMANENT INCISORS.

Among the differences that can be found between the primary and permanent dentition is the axis of the teeth. In primary teeth in general the interincisal angle between the upper and lower central incisors is about 150°, while in permanent incisors it is 123° (Fig. 37). The permanent incisors being much more labially inclined allow the dental arch to acquire a wider circumference, which benefits the positioning of the larger permanent incisors.

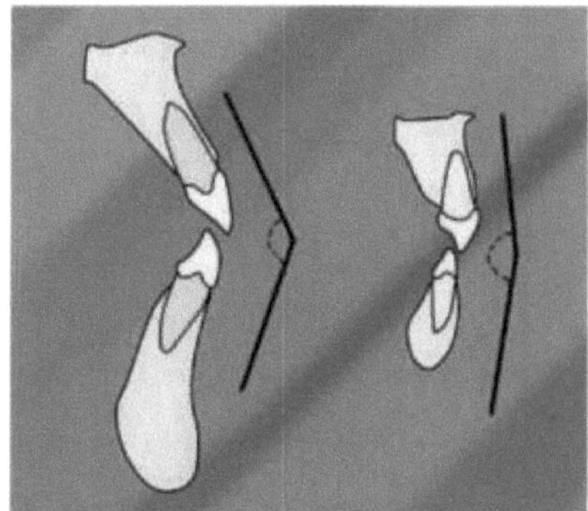

Fig. 37, Interincisal angle in primary and permanent dentition (Moyers 1992). Drawn by Castro E.

3) CHARACTERISTICS OF THE PERMANENT INCISORS DURING DENTITION

MIXED FIRST PHASE.

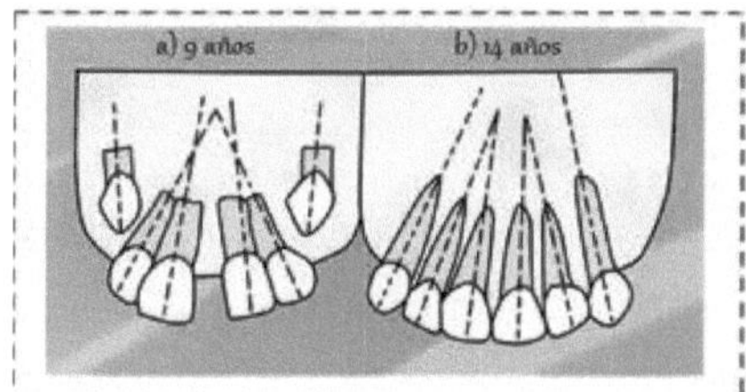

Fig. 38, Closure of diastema between permanent upper central incisors (Nakata 1992). Drawn by Castro E.

During incisor eruption children tend to look different, the permanent incisors are larger, their longitudinal axis is open in a reverse v-shape and the colour is more yellow in relation to the primary teeth (Fig. 38). The presence of diastema between the upper central incisors has been reported in 70% and spontaneous closure of the diastema in 82% of these cases. Due to the malalignment present at this time it has been called the "ugly duckling period". Subsequently the incisors will straighten out with the eruption of lateral incisors and canines

∧ 4) CONCEPT OF RESALT AND SCALOON

An important aspect of occlusion is the protrusion and stepping of the incisors, which can be defined as follows:

(A) HIGHLIGHTING, OVERJET OR HORIZONTAL PROJECTION:

The degree of protrusion in the permanent dentition depends on the permanent canine eruption and the anterior growth of the maxillary and mandibular arches. Its average value is 2.5 mm 5.

(B) STEP, OVERBITE OR VERTICAL PROJECTION:

In the permanent dentition the distance between the incisal edges vertically is on average 2.5 mm 5.

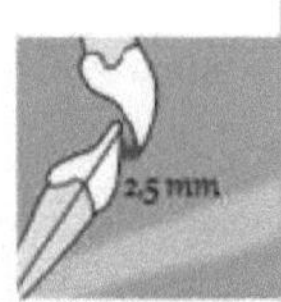

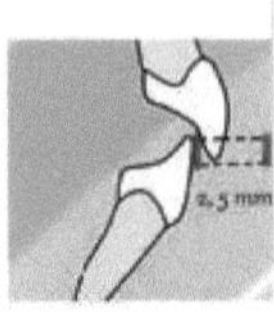

Fig. 39, Overjet. (Said 1992). Drawn by Castro E. Fig. 40, Overbite (Said 1992). Drawn by Castro E.

TEST OF THE THIRD UNIT

1. Which is the last tooth of the incisor group to initiate calcification according to Logan and Kronfeld?

a)   Upper lateral incisor.

b)   Lower lateral incisor.

c)   Upper central incisor.

d)   Lower central incisor.

2. Which is the first tooth of the incisor group to erupt according to Logan and Kronfeld?

a)   Upper lateral incisor.

b)   Lower lateral incisor.

c)   Upper central incisor.

d)   Lower central incisor.

3. What is the sum of the mesiodistal widths of permanent incisors in relation to that of primary incisors?

a)   Major.

b)   Similar.

c) Minor.

d) The same.

4. By how much is the increase in the intercanine width during the replacement of the incisors?

a)   7 mm in the upper jaw and 5 mm in the lower jaw.

b)   3 mm for each jaw.

c)   3 mm for upper jaw 1 mm for lower jaw.

d)   1 mm for each jaw.

5. Which of these factors facilitates the placement of permanent incisors?

a)   Anteriourdental augmentation.

b)   Mesial step.

c)   Physiological wear and tear.

d)   Molar field.

6. How is the axis of the permanent incisors in relation to the axis of the primary incisors?

a)   They are more inclined towards distai.

b)   They are more labially inclined.

c)   They are perpendicular to the occlusal plane.

d) They are more inclined mesially.

7. What is correct about the characteristics of the incisors during the first stage mixed dentition?

a) The permanent central incisors are converging mesially.

b) The primary incisors are more yellow in colour than the permanent incisors.

c) A diastema between the permanent central incisors is common and needs to be treated early.

d) A high percentage of the diastemas between the permanent central incisors close spontaneously.

8. What is the average value for overjet and overbite in permanent dentition?

a) 2.5 and 3mm respectively.

b) 1 mm for both.

c) 2.6 and 2.7 mm respectively.

d) 2.5 mm for both.

SOLUTIONS TO THE THIRD UNIT TEST

1. a) Upper lateral incisor.
2. (d) Lower central incisor.
3. a) Major.
4. (b) 3 mm for each jaw.
5. a) Anterior dental arch augmentation.
6. b) They are more labially inclined.
7. d) A high percentage of the diastemas between the permanent central incisors close spontaneously.
8. (d) 2,5 mm for both

REFERENCES

1. Boj J., Catalá M., García-Ballesta C., Mendoza A., Planells P. Odontopediatria, la evolución del niño al adulto joven. I⁰ Edicion. Madrid: RipanoS.A. 2011. P.81-84.

2. Pavic M., Cauvi D., Espinoza A. Characteristics of second stage mixed dentition in a sample of children in the metropolitan area. [Thesis for the degree of surgeon - dentist]. Santiago. University of Chile, Faculty of Dentistry, Dentomaxillary Orthopaedics. 1992. P. 3-4.

3. Buhn C., Hofrath H., Korkhaus G.. Orthodontics. 2° edition. Barcelona: Editorial Labor. 1934. P. 109 - 122.

4. Reichenbach E., Brückl H. Clinical and therapeutic orthopaedic - maxillary. I⁰ Edition. Argentina: Editorial Mundi. 1965. P. 21.

5. Said L., Cauvi. D., Espinoza A. Characteristics of mixed dentition I⁰ Phase in a population of Chilean children in the Metropolitan area. [Thesis for the degree of surgeon - dentist]. Santiago: Universidad de Chile, Facultad de Odontología, Asignatura de Ortopedia Dentomaxilar. 1992. P. 10-40, 75-78.

6. Leiva N., Cauvi D., Espinoza, A. Characteristics of the primary dentition in children between 6 and 24 months of age. [Thesis for the degree of Surgeon - Dentist]. Santiago: University of Chile, Faculty of Dentistry, Dentomaxillary Orthopaedics. 1994. P. 8-9.

7. Nakata M., Wei S. Guía Oclusal en Odontopediatria. 1st Edition, Venezuela: Actualidades medico odontologicas S.A. 1992. P. 14-21.

8. Rubio L., Cauvi D., Espinoza A. Characteristics of the normal primary dentition at the age of 5 years. Thesis for the degree of Surgeon - [Tesis para optar al título de Cirujano Dentist]. Santiago. University of Chile, Faculty of Dentistry, Subject of Dentomaxillary Orthopaedics. 1994. P. 4-7.

9. Pinto M. Anatomía dentaria evolución de la dentición. Practical Guide. University of Chile, Faculty of Dentistry, Subject of Paediatric Dentistry. 2013.

10. CanutJ. Clinical Orthodontics. 2° Edition. Barcelona: Ed Salvat. 2000. P. 49 - 55

11. Navarrete M., Cauvi D., Espinoza A. Characteristics of the normal primary dentition at 3 years of age. [Thesis for the degree of Surgeon - Dentist]. Santiago: University of Chile, Faculty of Dentistry, Dentomaxillary Orthopaedics. 1993. P. 18 -19.

12. Moyers R. Manual of orthodontics. 4° edition. Argentina: Editorial médica Panamericana. 1992. P.131-134.

CHAPTER 3

MIXED DENTITION SECOND PHASE.

> **Objectives**
>
> *By the end of this unit you will be able to explain:*
>
> *I.   The concept of mixed dentition second stage.*
>
> *II.   What is the Korkhaus Support Zone and what is its importance.*
>
> *III.   Which factors may affect the integrity of the Korkhaus Support Zone.*

I UNIT: RELEVANT CONCEPTS.

1) MIXED DENTITION SECOND STAGE

This stage begins with the replacement of the teeth that make up *the Korkhaus support zone* (Fig. 42), consisting of the canine, first and second primary molar, which are replaced by the permanent canine, first and second premolar, once the eruption of the permanent incisors is complete, approximately one and a half years later. The second stage mixed dentition develops *between 9 and 12 years of age* (Fig. 41).

During the one and a half year break after the eruption of the permanent incisors, the permanent canines and premolars will be placed in the appropriate position for their subsequent eruption and at the same time the roots of the primary teeth will be gradually resorbed, and at this time the formation and calcification of the roots of all permanent teeth will also take place.

Although molar occlusion is largely determined in the period of mixed dentition first phase, with the eruption of the first permanent molars, the knowledge of how the replacement of the teeth in the lateral areas takes place is of great importance as occlusal abnormalities can manifest themselves in a constant or more or less pronounced manner ≡.

2) KORKHAUS SUPPORT ZONE (KSK) AND ITS IMPORTANCE.

The Korkhaus Support Zone is the area between mesial of the primary canine and distai of the second primary molar, and its function is to accommodate permanent canines and premolars. It consists of the canine, first and second molar.

primary

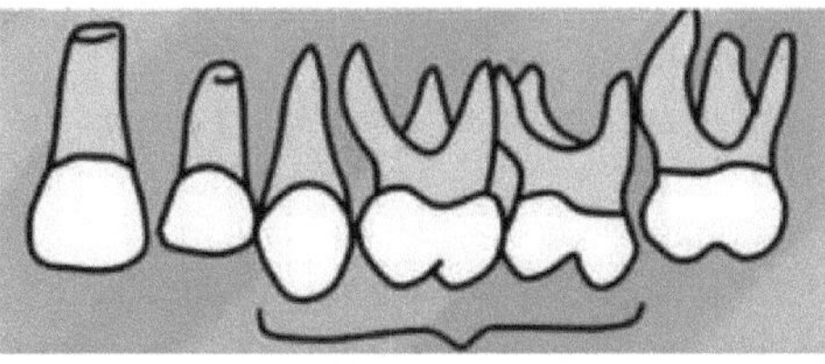

ZSK

Fig. 42, Korkhaus Support Zone (Álvarez 1995). Drawn by Castro E.

The importance of the Korkhaus Holding Zone is manifested during the first stage mixed dentition by maintaining the occlusion in the three directions of space: it maintains the height and gearing of the occlusion and preserves the space that canines and premolars will occupy by maintaining the perimeter of the dental arch K

If the Z.S.K. maintains its integrity, then normal tooth replacement will take place, however, it can be affected by various factors, which can affect its integrity, leading to alterations in tooth replacement к

(c) FACTORS AFFECTING THE INTEGRITY OF THE KORKHAUS SUPPORT ZONE

❖ *CARIES:* When a dental caries located interproximally to the teeth generates a loss of tissue, a zone of lower resistance is generated to which neighbouring teeth will migrate and invade the ZSK.

❖ *AGENESIAS* : this can be assumed when the period between the exfoliation of the primary tooth and the eruption of the permanent tooth is longer than 2 months.

❖ *EARLY LOSS OF A PRIMARY TOOTH:* Early loss of a primary tooth either by early extraction or trauma, as in the case of caries, generates an area of reduced resistance to which neighbouring teeth will migrate and invade the ZSK.

❖ *PREVIOUS ZSK ATTACK:* Occurs when there is premature rhizalysis of the primary canines with or without loss of the primary canine K

❖ *POSTERIOR ZSK ATTACK:* This is caused by the malposition of the eruption of the first permanent molar, which follows a too mesial route, which will cause difficulty to emerge and will cause damage to the root of the second primary molar. The mesial position of the permanent molar will mean that the dental arch is crowded.

TEST OF THE FIRST UNIT

1. At approximately what age does the Second Stage Mixed Dentition develop?
a) Between 5.5 and 9 years.
b) Between 9 and 2 years.
c) Between 9 and 5 years.
d) Between 5.5 and 2.5 years.
2. What is the Korkhaus Support Zone?
a) The area from mesial of the primary canine to distal of the second primary molar.
b) The area from distal of the primary canine to mesial of the second primary molar.
c) Area comprising the permanent canine, first and second premolars.
d) The area from mesial of the primary lateral incisor to distal of the primary second molar.
3. What is the function of the Korkhaus Holding Zone?
a) To allow neutroclusion of the second permanent molar.
b) To allow preservation of the postlacteal plane.
c) To allow the first physiological raising of the first permanent molar.
d) Maintain occlusion in all three directions of space.
4. Which of the following factors can affect the integrity of the Korkhaus Support Zone?
a) Presence of incipient caries.
b) Presence of impacted third molars.
c) CorrimientoTardio.
d) Presence of scalondistal.

5. Why does the Korkhaus Holding Area Subsequent Attack occur?

a) Due to premature rhizalysis of the primary canine.

b) Eruption of the second permanent molar before the second premolar.

c) Due to the absence of one of the permanent teeth that will be located in the Korkhaus Support area.

d) Damage to the root of the primary second molar.

SOLUTIONS TO THE FIRST UNIT TEST

1. b) Between 9 and 2 years of age.
2. (a) Area from mesial of primary canine to distal of second primary molar.
3. (d) Maintain occlusion in all three directions of space.
4. (c) Late Run-up.
5. (d) Damage to the root of the second primary molar.

UNIT II: DEVELOPMENT OF THE MIXED DENTITION SECOND STAGE.

Objectives

By the end of this unit you will be able to explain:

I.   *How the development* and *chronology of eruption of permanent canines* and *premolars takes place.*

II. *What is drift space, Nance free space or Lee WaySpace.*

III. *How the development* and *eruption of the second permanent molar takes place.*

1) DEVELOPMENT AND ERUPTION OF CANINES AND PREMOLARS.

The upper and lower permanent canines begin hard tissue formation between 4 to 5 months of age, while their finished enamel is visible between 6 to 7 years of age. The lower permanent canines erupt first between 9 and 10 years of age and then the upper permanent canines erupt between 10 and 11 years of age (Table 7).

As for the first premolars, the upper premolars begin hard tissue formation at one and a half years and the lower premolars at one year and 9 months. Both complete their enamel formation between 5 and 6 years of age. The upper first premolar erupts between 10 and 11 years of age and the lower first premolar erupts between 10 and 12 years of age 5.

The upper second premolars begin hard tissue formation at about 2 years of age and the lower second premolars at 2 years and 3 months. Both complete their enamel formation between 6 and 7 years of age. The upper second premolar erupts between 10 and 12 years of age and the lower second premolar between 11 and 12 years of age 5. The chronology used by the Paediatric Dentistry Department of the Faculty of Dentistry of the University of Chile θ is also attached (Table 8).

TABLE 7: Chronology of the development of the Permanent Dentition according to					
Teeth	Home training fabric hard	Quantity from enamel at birth	Enamele ends do	Eruption	Root finished
Superio					
Canine	4-5 months	-	6-7 years	11-12 years	13-15 years
I⁰ PM	1½-1 ¾ years	-	5-6 years	10 -11 years	12-13 years
2⁰ PM	2-2% years	-	6-7 years	10-12 years	12 -14years
Inferior					
Canine	4-5	-	6-7	9-10	12-14
I⁰ PMI	I¾-a2 years	-	5-6 years	10-12 years	12-13 years
2⁰ PMI	2%-2 ½ years	-	6-7 years	11-12 years	13-14 years

TABLE8: Eruption chronology in Permanent Dentition used by		
Teeth Permanent	*Maxilla (years)*	*Mandible (years)*
Canines	11-12	9-11
I⁰ Premolar	10-11	10-12
2⁰ Premolar	10-12	12 -13

The space for the eruption of these teeth is rather limited, therefore some conditions must exist for a gradual eruption of the permanent canines and premolars to take place. These are mentioned below[7] .

A) NANCE FREE SPACE OR LEE WAY SPACE.

It corresponds to the space generated by the difference of the sum of the mesiodistal widths of primary canines and molars in relation to that of permanent canines and premolars, which is smaller, the difference being approximately 1 mm in the maxilla and approximately 3 mm in the mandible[7] (Fig.43).

If each tooth is analysed, the permanent canine is larger than the primary, the first premolar is smaller than the first primary molar and the second premolar is smaller than the second primary premolar, thus creating crowding as each tooth changes, which is related to the change in order of the teeth in the lateral segment. The loss of space eventually resolves by exfoliating the second primary molar[7] .

Thanks to the existence of the nance free space, cases in which the terminal plane is vertical and without spaces in the primary dental arch, where the occlusion of the first permanent molars is in a cuspid-cuspid relationship, can be transformed into Class I, through the mesial displacement of the first permanent lower molars, during the replacement of the teeth of the ZSK. On the other hand, a crowding in the anterior sector after lateral incisor replacement can be relieved by the existence of this space 7

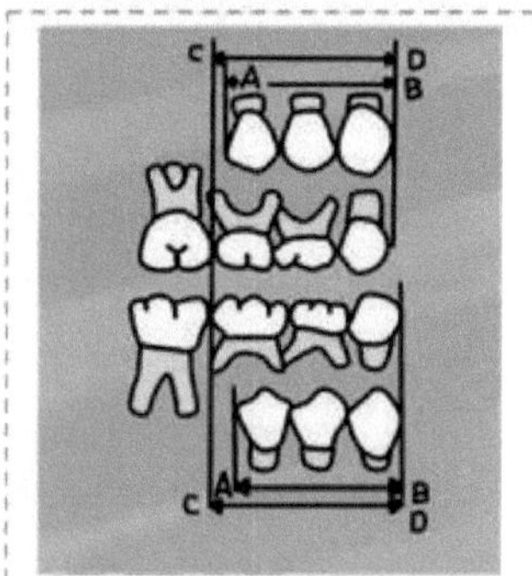

Fig. 43, Nance's Free Space (Nakata 1992). Drawn by Castro E.

B)   ORDER OF CHANGING THE SIDE TEETH.

The order of change of the lateral teeth is an important factor, because it develops in a short time, under difficult conditions and in limited space in the dental arch Λ.

The order of eruption of canines and premolars is carried out in order to achieve an adequate interlocking, which is why it is done in a logical manner. The sequence is different for the maxilla and mandible and according to sex, since in girls it starts half a year to a year earlier.

Tooth eruption takes about *two and a half years.* In this period of the dentition there is considerable variation in the sequence of eruption of canines and premolars κ

The most favourable sequence for the upper jaw (Fig. 44), according to most authors, is:

1.   1st FP → 2nd FP → Canine → 2nd M

2.   1st PM → Canine → 2nd PM → 2nd M K

In both sequences after the eruption of the first premolar, which is generally not difficult as it is similar in size to the first primary molar, there is a pause of approximately one year, during which the primary canine is exfoliated and the permanent canine prepares for its eruption, this tooth follows a more tortuous path, so that the second premolar, which usually has a more direct location, erupts before the canine.

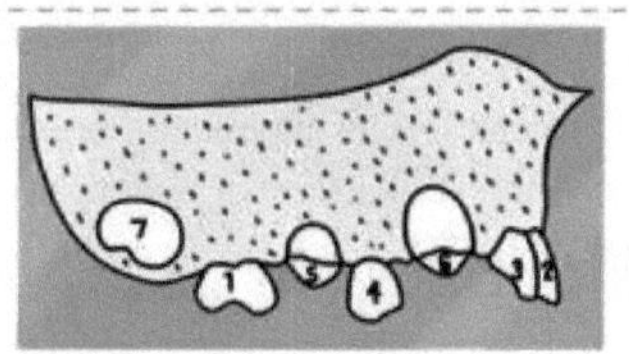

Fig. 44, Eruption sequence in the upper jaw (Pavic 1992). Drawn by Castro E.

Some authors point out that during the eruption of the canine, the second primary molar is lost, which allows the first premolar to move distally by 2 mm, giving free space to the permanent canine, which requires more space. Other authors agree on the existence of the distal movement of the first premolar and point out that

that the canines fit better in the arch when erupting simultaneously with the second premolars к

The most common and favourable sequence for the lower jaw (Fig. 45), according to most authors is:

1.   Canine $\rightarrow$ 1st FP $\rightarrow$ 2nd FP $\rightarrow$ 2nd M

It is feasible to find two more sequences with some frequency, which are:

2.   Canine $\rightarrow$ 1erPM $\rightarrow$ 2nd M $\rightarrow$ 2nd PM

3.   1erPM $\rightarrow$ Canine $\rightarrow$ 2ndPM $\rightarrow$ 2nd M к

In half of the cases, the lower canine erupts before the lower premolars, which is beneficial as it helps to maintain the length of the dental arch and avoids the lingual inclination of the lower premolars.

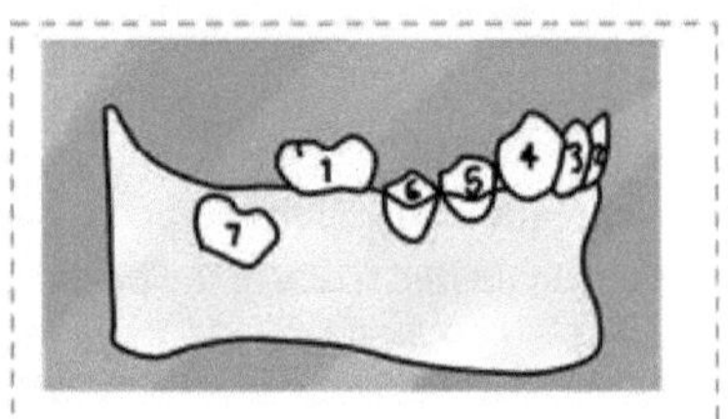

Fig. 45, Eruption sequence in the lower jaw (Pavic 1992). Drawn by Castro

incisors θ. When the root development of the canine is more rapid, it can be positioned slightly before the first premolar in the dental arch θ>.

As for the second premolar there is considerable variation in its development. However, it usually erupts on both dental arches at the same time θ>.

On the other hand, it has been described that there are differences in the eruption sequences between the two sexes, which are shown below:

CHILDREN

- Canine 1erPM $\rightarrow$ $\rightarrow$ 2ndPM $\rightarrow$ 2ndM

- Canine 1erPM $\rightarrow$ $\rightarrow$ 2ndM $\rightarrow$ 2ndPM GIRLS

- Canine $\rightarrow$ 1erPM 2ndPM 2ndM $\rightarrow$ $\rightarrow$

- 1erPM $\rightarrow$ Canine 2ndPM $\rightarrow$ $\rightarrow$ 2ndM

In boys there is a constant sequence between canine and first premolar, while there is a difference in the second premolar and second molar, whereas in girls there is a constant sequence between second premolar and second molar and the difference is found in the canine and first premolar K

2) DEVELOPMENT AND ERUPTION OF THE SECOND PERMANENT MOLAR.

The upper second permanent molar starts its hard tissue formation at about 2.5 to 3 months, the lower second permanent molar at about 2.5 to 3 years. Both complete their enamel formation between 7 and 8 years of age. The upper lower second molar erupts between the ages of 11 and 13 years, while the upper second molar erupts between the ages of 12 and 13 years (Table 9). The chronology of eruption of the second permanent molar used by the paediatric dentistry department of the Faculty of Dentistry of the University of Chile θ is attached (Table 9).

TABLE9:	Developmental chronology of the permanent dentition according to Logan and Kronfeld, slightly modified by McCall and Schour 5.				
Teeth	Home hard tissue formation	Amount of enamel at birth	Finished enamel	Eruption	Finished root
2° MS	2½A3 months	-	7-8 years	12 -13 years	14-16 years
2° MI	2½a3 years	-	7-8 years	11-13 years	14-15 years

TABLE 10: Chronology of eruption in the Permanent Dentition used by		
Teeth Permanent	Maxilla (years)	Mandible (years)
2° Molar	12 14	
3° Molar	17 30	

When the shifting of the lateral segment teeth has been completed and the dental arch has been established from the first permanent molar, the second permanent molars begin to erupt. Prior to eruption, in most cases, the length of the dental arch will be reduced by eruptive forces mesial to the second permanent molar. Generally with the eruption of this tooth, the circumference of the arch becomes smaller than that of the primary arch, due to the use of the drifting space, so it is possible to find an accentuated crowding depending on the sequence and conditions of tooth replacement. On the other hand, caries and premature extractions of the primary second molar will cause an additional loss of space, which will affect the eruption and relationship of the molar region. Finally there are cases where the second permanent molar erupts before the second premolar, in these cases the space of the unerupted tooth must be maintained otherwise it will be lost.

TEST OF THE SECOND UNIT

1. Between what ages do permanent canines erupt according to Logan and Kronfeld?
a) Between the ages of 9yll.
b) Between the ages of 2 years and 2 years.

c)   Between 9 and 5 years old

d)   Between 1 and 2 years.

2.   What is Nance's free space?

a)   The area between the canine, first and second primary molar.

b)   Space generated by the greater mesiodistal width of primary canines and molars in relation to permanent canines and premolars.

c)   This is the space where the permanent canine and premolars are located.

d)   Refers to the physiological spaces located mesial and distai to the primary upper and lower canine respectively.

3.   Is the replacement of the Korkhaus Support Zone correct?

a)   The replacement sequence is the same for both sexes.

b)   TomacercadeS years.

c)   The sequence is different between jaws and according to sex.

d)   The order of tooth replacement is not an important factor.

4.   What is the most favourable eruption sequence of the maxillary lateral segment?

a)   1st PM ÷ Canine ÷ 2nd PM ÷ 2nd M

b)   Canine ÷ 1st PM ÷ 2nd PM ÷ 2nd M

c)   Canine ÷ IerPM ÷ 2nd M ÷ 2nd PM

d)   1st PM ÷ 2nd PM ÷Canino ÷ 2nd M

5.   What is the most favourable eruption sequence of the maxillary lateral segment?

a)   1st PM ÷ Canine ÷ 2nd PM ÷ 2nd M

b)   Canine ÷ 1st PM ÷ 2nd PM ÷ 2nd M

c)   Canine ÷ IerPM ÷ 2nd M ÷ 2nd PM

d)   1st PM ÷ 2nd PM ÷Canino ÷ 2nd M

6.   Why is it beneficial to erupt the lower permanent canine before the premolars and lower second molar?

a)   Because it maintains the length of the arch and prevents lingual inclination of the permanent incisors.

b)   Because it allows the neutroclusion of the first permanent molar to be generated.

c)   Because it prevents tilting of the Kaciavestibular permanent incisors.

d)   Because it maintains the space for the eruption of the first permanent molar.

7.   At what age does calcification of the second permanent molar end?

a)   Between 2 and 3 years.

b)   Between 2 and 3 years.

c)   Between 7 and 8 years.

d)   Between the years.

1. a) Between 9yll years of age.

2. b) Space generated by the greater mesiodistal width of primary canines and molars in relation to permanent canines and premolars.

3. c) The sequence is different between jaws and according to sex.

4. d) 1st MP ÷ 2nd MP ÷Canine ÷ 2nd M

5. b) Canine ÷ 1st MP ÷ 2nd MP ÷ 2nd M

6. a) Because it maintains the length of the arch and avoids the lingual inclination of the permanent incisors.

7. (c) Between 7 and 8 years.

III UNIT: DETERMINANTS OF OCCLUSION.

> ***Objectives***
> *By the end of this unit you will be able to explain:*
> *I.	The importance of the mesiodistal diameter of laZSK.*
> *II.	The methods used to determine the mesiodistal diameter of laZSK.*
> *III.	The determinants of occlusion.*
> *IV.	General and local factors can affect occlusal determinants.*

1) IMPORTANCE OF MESIO-DISTAL DIAMETER

The mesiodistal diameter of the Z.S.K. is of great importance both in the first stage mixed dentition and in the second stage mixed dentition, due to the fact that during the replacement of primary teeth by permanent teeth it undergoes dimensional alterations ⅛ θ. Several authors have pointed out that the perimeter of the dental arch decreases from the end of the primary dentition until the permanent dentition, and it has also been described that the decrease is greater in girls than in boys and stabilises after the age of 14 years in both sexes.

The shortening of the arch perimeter is often attributed to the eruption of the first permanent molar, which would generate a mesial shift that closes the existing physiological spaces (diastemas, the drifting space) K

2) METHODS FOR DETERMINING THE MESIO-DISTAL DIAMETER.

In order to achieve an adequate diagnosis and management of the mesiodistal diameter of canines and premolars prior to their eruption, it is necessary to know methods that allow us to estimate with certain precision this κ value.

Three main parameters are used for this purpose:

1. Direct measurement of the width of permanent canines and premolars on radiographs.

2. By means of the Moyers' Index.

3. By means of theTanakaH.

Moyers' index: This is the ratio between the sum of the mesiodistal diameters of the four lower incisors and the sum of the diameters that the permanent canine and premolars should have. It is obtained by applying the lower incisor sum to the Moyers table, which gives values for canines and premolars. Usually the table is used with a 75th percentile, which means that it is valid for 75% of the cases (see table).

Tanaka index: It is the ratio between the lower incisor sum and the space needed to place the permanent canine and the premolars, applying the following formula.

UPPER MAXILLARY= (lower incisor sum) + 11 mm
2

This determines the space for the permanent canine and upper premolars on one side.

LOWER MAXILLARY= (sum of lower incisor) + 10.5 mm 2

Which determines the space for permanent canine and lower premolars on one side.

TABLE 11: Moyers index [11]		
Lower incisor sum	Upper jaw	Lower jaw
19,5	20,6	20,1
20	20,9	20,4
20,5	21,2	20,7
21	21,5	21
21,5	21,8	21,3
22	22	21,6
22,5	22,3	21,9
23	22,6	22,2
23,5	22,9	22,5
24	23,1	22,8
24,5	23,4	23,1
25	23,7	23,4
25,5	24	23,7
26	24,2	24
26,5	24,5	24,3
27	24,8	24,6
27,5	25	24,8
28	25,3	25,1
28,5	25,6	25,4
29	25,9	25,7

3) DETERMINANTS OF OCCLUSION

The favourable development of occlusion depends on four factors, namely:

1. Favourable eruption sequence.

2. Satisfactory tooth size to space ratio.

3. To achieve a normal molar relationship, with minimal decrease in space available for premolars.

4. Favourable vestibulo-lingual relationship of the alveolar processes K

Given that the first three factors have been mentioned throughout the handbook

We will describe the last point.

A) VESTIBULO-LINGUAL RELATIONSHIP

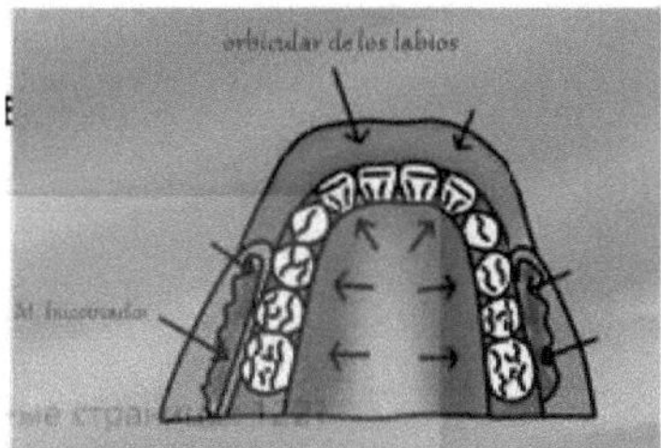

Fig. 46, Diagram of the forces exerted on the dental arches (Graber 1965). Drawn

The teeth are located between different muscle groups. Intraorally there are the tongue muscles and extraorally there are the orbicularis oris and buccinator in the cheek.

The forces exerted by these muscles on the teeth must be balanced in such a way as to allow them to be positioned correctly in relation to the lingual vestibule/palate.

When one or more of the above-mentioned determinants of occlusion are not fulfilled either by general or local factors, dental eruption and occlusion will be impaired к

4) GENERAL FACTORS AFFECTING OCCLUSAL DETERMINANTS

a)   Genetics.

b)   Prepubertal endocrine factors. Influence the difference in tooth eruption between the sexes, which is from 3 to 11 months earlier in girls.

c)   Race.

d)   Diet

e)   Infectious diseases and acute febrile processes. Delay the age of eruption.

f)   Climate.

g)   Constitutional types.

h)   Social status. Some studies have indicated that lower social levels have somewhat delayed tooth replacement к

5) LOCAL FACTORS AFFECTING OCCLUSAL DETERMINANTS.

a)   Caries.

b)   Persistence of primary teeth.

c)   Local conditions in the dental arches. Such as trauma or bad habits.

d)   Lack of germ or aberrant development of the permanent tooth K

TEST OF THE THIRD UNIT

1.   To what is the shortening of the dental arch attributed after completion of the primary dentition?

a)   At the eruption of the first permanent molar.

b)   To the replacement of the ZSK.

c)   The influence of endocrine factors.

d)   To the eruptive force of the permanent canine.

2.   Which of the following methods can be used to determine the mesiodistal diameter of permanent canines and premolars prior to eruption?

a)   Measurement of the width of permanent canines and premolars in plaster models.

b)   Measurement of the width of primary canines and molars on radiographs.

c) Measurement of the width of permanent canines and premolars on radiographs.

d) Measurement of the width of permanent canines and molars in plaster models.

3. How is the Moyers index obtained?

a) Applying the lower incisor sum to a table that gives values for canines and premolars according to jaw.

b) Establishing the relationship between the lower incisor sum and the space needed to place the permanent canine and premolars, according to a formula.

c) Measuring the mesiodistal width of the permanent canine and premolars on an X-ray.

d) Measuring the mesiodistal width of the permanent canine and premolars on a plaster cast.

4. How is the Tanaka index obtained?

a) Applying the lower incisor sum to a table that gives values for canines and premolars according to jaw.

b) Establishing the relationship between the lower incisor sum and the space needed to place the permanent canine and premolars, according to a formula.

c) Measuring the mesiodistal width of the permanent canine and premolars on an X-ray.

d) Measuring the mesiodistal width of the permanent canine and premolars on a plaster model.

5. Which of the following is a determinant of occlusion?

a) Relationship of the distal surfaces of primary second molars.

b) Angle class.

c) Skeletal Class.

d) Favourable sequence of eruption.

6. On what does it depend whether a favourable vestibulo-lingual relationship of the teeth is achieved?

a) That the forces exerted by the muscles lingual to the teeth are greater than those exerted vestibular to the teeth.

b) That the forces exerted by the muscles lingual to the teeth are less than those exerted vestibular to them.

c) That there are no forces acting on the teeth.

d) That the forces exerted by the lingual and vestibular muscles of the teeth are balanced.

7. What general factor can affect occlusal determinants?

a) Caries.

b) Persistence of primary teeth.

c) Genetics.

d) Bad habits.

SOLUTIONS TO THE THIRD UNIT TEST

1. (a) At the eruption of the first permanent molar.

2. c) Measurement of the width of permanent canines and premolars on radiographs.

3. a) Applying the lower incisor sum to a table that gives values for canines and premolars according to jaw.

4. b) Establishing the relationship between the lower incisor sum and the space needed to place the permanent canine and the premolars, according to a formula.

5.   d) Favourable eruption sequence.

6.   d) That the forces exerted by the lingual and vestibular muscles of the teeth are balanced.

7.   c) Genetics.

REFERENCES

1. Pavic M., Cauvi D., Espinoza A. Characteristics of second stage mixed dentition in a sample of children in the metropolitan area. [Thesis for the degree of surgeon - dentist]. Santiago. University of Chile, Faculty of Dentistry, Dentomaxillary Orthopaedics. 1992. P.4-30, 81 - 83.

2. Hotz R., Rinderer L., Stöckli P., Ben - Zur E. Orthodontics in daily practice 2nd Edition. Spain: Editorial Científico. Médica. 1974. P. 36-45.

3. Mayoral J., Mayoral G., GraberT. Orthodontics: Fundamental Principles and Practice. 3° Edition. Barcelona: Editorial Labor. 1977. P. 57-68.

4. Proffit W., Fields H. Sarver D. Contemporary Orthodontics. 4° Edition. Spain: Elsevier. 2008. P. 139.

5. Boj J., Catalá M., García-Ballesta C., Mendoza A., Planells P. Odontopediatria, la evolución del niño al adulto joven. I⁰ Edicion. Madrid: RipanoS.A. 2011. P.81-84.

6. Pinto M. Anatomía dentaria evolución de la dentición. Practical Guide. University of Chile, Faculty of Dentistry, Subject of Paediatric Dentistry. 2013.

7. Nakata M., Wei S. Guía Oclusal en Odontopediatria. I⁰ Edition, Venezuela: Actualidades medico odontologicas S.A. 1992. P.22 -23.

8. Moyers R. "Manual de Ortodoncia" 4° Edition. Argentina:Editorial médica Panamericana. 1992. P. 139 - 142.

9. Bruhn C., Hofrath H., Korkhaus G. Orthodontics. 2° edition. Volume IV. Barcelona: Editorial Labor. 1944. P. 122 -140.

10. Braham R., Morris M. Paediatric Dentistry. I⁰ Edition. Buenos Aires: Editorial médica Panamericana. 1984. P. 383-385.

11. Bustamante S., Cauvi D. " Analysis of models for orthopaedics and Orthodontics". SantiagoiUniversity of Chile, Faculty of Dentistry, Department of Child and Dentomaxillary Orthopaedics, Dentomaxillary Area. P. 26-29.

12. GraberT-M-Orthodontics: Principles and Practice. I⁰ Edicion-Argentina: EditorialMundi. 1965. P. 88 - 91.

FINAL TEST

1. In which week do facial prominences appear?
a) G^0 Semanadevidenceintrauterine.
b) S^0 Semanadevidenceintrauterine.
c) 4th month of intrauterine life.
d) 4th week of intrauterine life.

2. What structure is formed from the junction of the medial nasal and maxillary maxillary prominences?
a) Fossa nasalis.
b) Coanasprimitives.
c) Labiosuperior.
d) Palatine ridges.

3. Which teeth contain the "palatal component" of the intermaxillary segment?
a) Upper canine and incisors.
b) Lower incisors.
c) Premolars and upper molars.
d) Upper incisors.

4. Between which week(s) can we find "embryonic progeny"?
a) During the tenth week of intrauterine life.
b) From the eleventh to the twelfth week of intrauterine life.
c) From the twelfth week of intrauterine life until birth.
d) During the twelfth week of intrauterine life.

5. At what stage of odontogenesis do papilla cells differentiate into odontoblasts?
a) EtapadeYema.
b) Bonnet Stage.
c) Campana Stage.
d) Dental film stage.

6. When does the germ formation of primary teeth begin?
a) 4^0 weekintrauterinelife.
b) 4^0 monthintrauterinelife.
c) G^0 Semanadevidenceintrauterine.
d) 6^0 monthintrauterinelife.

7. What are suction impellers?
a) Fibrous cord located in the occlusal region of incisors and canines.
b) Radial prominences located at the level of the lips.
c) Segmented structures overlying the alveolar processes.
d) Prominences located on both sides of the palate.

8. What could a "Box Top Occlusion" evolve into according to Schwarz?
a) Covered Bite.
b) Open bite.
c) Crossbite.
d) Crowding.

9. What is the position of the tooth germs inside the jaws between 0 and 5 months of age?

a) Aligned.

b) Crowded and staggered.

c) Rotated.

d) Staggered.

10. what is the level of calcification of the first primary molar at birth?

a) Crown almost entirely calcified.

b) Two thirds of the crown calcified.

c) One third of the crown calcified.

d) Vertex of mesiovestibular cusp calcified.

11. What happens during the first phase of breastfeeding?

a) The mandible descends and a vacuum is formed in the anterior region, with the posterior region remaining closed.

b) The first physiological advancement of the occlusion is generated.

c) The tongue takes the form of a spoon.

d) The lower jaw slides forward.

12. What is "dental emergency"?

a) The time when the tooth is present in the mouth without making contact with its antagonist.

b) It is the intra-alveolar migration of the tooth.

c) When the tooth perforates the gingiva but is no more than 3 mm visible.

d) The moment when the tooth begins its movement into the oral cavity.

13. When does the first physiological lifting of the occlusion occur?

a) With the eruption of the first four permanent molars.

b) With the eruption of the four second permanent molars.

c) With the eruption of the first primary molars.

d) With the eruption and occlusion of the first four primary molars.

14. At what age is the primary dentition fully erupted?

a) At 6 months of age.

b) At 2 years of age.

c) At 2.5 years of age.

d) At 6 years of age.

15. How does mandibular-sagittal growth take place?

a) By distai bone apposition and mesial resorption of the ascending branches of the mandible.

b) By apposition in the area of the tuberosity.

c) By distai resorption and mesial apposition of the mandibular ramus.

d) By internal apposition and internal resorption of the mandibular body.

16. What is the step and step at 2 years of age?

a) 2, 5 mm for both.

b) 2.6 and 2.7 mm respectively.

c) Imm for both.

d) 0.5ylmm respectively.

17. What does the implantation of primary teeth look like at 3 years of age?

a) Perpendicular to the occlusal plane.

b) They have a kaciavestibular inclination.

c) They present a physiological overbite.

d) The anteroinferior teeth are lingually inclined.

18. What is the occlusal contact relationship like at 3 years of age?

a) Occlusal-physiological wear is present.

b) There is a sharp gear.

c) There is a weak cusp - fossa relationship.

d) Primate spaces are present.

19. What is the "molar field"?

a) That the distal faces of primary second molars are in the same vertical plane.

b) That the distal faces of primary first molars are in the same vertical plane.

c) 9 mm space distal to the second primary molars.

d) Space that will allow the eruption of the first primary molar.

20. What is the occlusal contact relationship like at 5 years of age?

a) There is a sharp gearing, due to the cusp-fossa relationship.

b) Physiological spaces are present.

c) There is little pronounced gearing, due to physiological wear and tear.

d) the presence of postlacteal plane, mesial step or distai can be observed.

21. Between what ages does the Mixed Dentition I^0 Phase develop?

a) 5.5 to 9 years old.

b) 5 to 9 years of age.

c) 6 to 0 years of age.

d) 9 to 2 years of age.

22. When does organogenesis of the first permanent molar begin?

a) 4° monthIntrauterine life

b) 6^0 monthintrauterinelife.

c) 7^0 monthintrauterinelife.

d) 4^0 weekintrauterinelife.

23. What is the direction of eruption of the upper first permanent molar?

a) Downwards and backwards.

b) Upwards and backwards.

c) Downwards and forwards.

d) Downwards and towards the vestibular.

24. Which of these mechanisms achieves neutroclusion of the permanent first molar from a postlacteal plane relationship?

a) Mesial advancement of the mandible.

b) First physiological breakthrough.

c) Second physiological relevance.

d) Mesial step.

25. At what age does the eruption of the permanent lower central incisor occur according to Logan and Kronfeld?

a) Between 8 and 9 years old.

b) Between 6 and 7 years
c) Between 7 and 8 years old.
d) Between 9 and 10 years old.
26. Why does anterior arch augmentation occur during incisor replacement?
a) Because permanent incisors have a sharper axis of implantation than primary incisors.
b) The presence of physiological spaces in the primary dentition.
c) For the more labial eruption of the permanent incisors, 2 to 3 mm in relation to the primary incisors.
d) The appearance of the diastema between the permanent central incisors during their eruption.
27. What is the definition of mixed dentition $2°$ phase?
a) Phase that develops between 5 and 9 years of age, where primary and permanent teeth are present.
b) Condition in which both primary and permanent teeth can be observed in the mouth.
c) Phase from 9 to 12 years of age when the first molar and permanent incisors erupt.
d) Stage that begins with the replacement of the teeth in the support area of the Korkhaus and ranges from 9 to 12 years.
28. Which teeth make up the Korkhaus support zone?
a) Canine and permanent and permanent and permanent molars.
b) Canine and primary molars.
c) Lateral incisor, canine and primary molar.
d) Lateral incisor, canine and permanent molar.
29. At what age does the first upper premolar erupt according to Logan and Kronfeld?
a) lOyll years
b) 10yl2years
c) llyl2years
d) 13yl4years.
30. What is "Lee way Space"?
a) Space distal to the second primary molars.
b) Spaces distal to the upper primary canine and distal to the lower primary canine.
c) Space generated by the difference in the sum of the mesiodistal widths of primary canines and molars in relation to permanent canines and premolars.
d) Space created between the permanent central incisors during eruption.
31. What is correct about the teeth that are located in the Korkhaus Support Zone?
a) The second premolar is larger than the second primary molar.
b) The permanent canine is smaller than the primary canine.
c) The permanent canine is the same size as the primary canine.
d) The first premolar is similar in size to the first primary molar.
32. What is the sequence of eruption of the lateral segment in the maxilla?
a) First premolar, second premolar, canine and second permanent molar.
b) Second premolar, first premolar, canine and second permanent molar.
c) Canine, first premolar, second premolar and second permanent molar.
d) Second premolar, first premolar, second permanent molar and canine.

33. What is the most favourable eruption sequence of the lateral segment for
jaw?
a)   Canine, second, premolar, first premolar and second molar.
b)   Canine, first premolar, second premolar and second molar.
c)   First premolar, second premolar, canine and second molar.
d)   Second molar, canine, first premolar, second premolar.
34. At what age does the enamel of the second permanent molar finish forming according
to Logan and Kronfeld?
a)   12 to 13 years old
b)   2 to 3 years
c)   7 to 8 years
d)   14 to 16 years.
35. What does the Moyers and Tanaka index measure?
a)   The lower incisor sum
b)   The mesiodistal diameter of primary canines and molars.
c)   The mesiodistal diameter of permanent canines and molars.
d)   The mesiodistal diameter of permanent canines and premolars, prior to eruption.
36. Which local factor affects occlusal determinants?
a)   Trauma.
b)   Genetics.
c)   Diet.
d) Constitutional types.

1. (c) 4th month of intrauterine life.
2. (c) Upper lip.
3. (d) Upper incisors.
4. (b) From the eleventh to the twelfth week of intrauterine life.
5. c) Campana Stage.
6. c) $6°$ week of intrauterine life.
7. b) Radial prominences located at the level of the lips.
8. a) Covered Bite.
9. a) Aligned.
10. c) One third of the crown calcified.
11. a) The mandible descends and a vacuum is formed in the anterior region and the posterior region remains closed.
12. (c) When the tooth perforates the gingiva but is not more than 3 mm visible.
13. d) With the eruption and occlusion of the first four primary molars.
14. (c) At 2.5 years of age.
15. a) By distai bone apposition and mesial resorption of the ascending branches of the mandible.
16. c) Imm for both.
17. (a) Perpendicular to the occlusal plane.
18. b) There is a sharp gear.
19. (c) 9 mm space distal to the second primary molars.
20. c) There is little pronounced gearing, due to physiological wear and tear. 21.a) 5.5 to 9 years of age.
22. a)$4°$ monthIntrauterine life
23. a) Downwards and backwards.
24. a) Mesial advancement of the mandible.
25. (b) Between 6 and 7 years
26. c) By the more labial eruption of the permanent incisors, 2 to 3 mm in relation to the primary incisors.
27. d) Stage beginning with the replacement of the teeth of the Korkhaus Supporting Zone and ranging from 9 to 12 years of age.
28. b) Canine and primary molars.
29. b) 10 and 12 years
30. c) Space generated by the difference of the sum of the mesiodistal widths of primary canines and molars in relation to permanent canines and premolars.
31. d) The first premolar is of a similar size to the first primary molar.
32. a) First premolar, second premolar, canine and second permanent molar.
33. (b) Canine, first premolar, second premolar and second molar.
34. c)7 to 8 years
35. d) The mesiodistal diameter of permanent canines and premolars, prior to eruption.
36. a) Trauma.

1) DEVELOPMENT AND ERUPTION OF THE PERMANENT INCISORS.

According to Logan and Kronfeld's chronology, modified by McCall and Schour, both the upper and lower central incisors and the lower lateral incisors show their first evidence of calcification 3 to 4 months after birth. On the other hand, the upper lateral incisors begin to calcify at approximately 10 to 12 months of age. The calcification of the eight permanent incisors is completed between 4 and 5 years of age K

As for their eruption, according to the chronology used by Logan and Kronfeld modified by McCall and Schour (Table 5), it occurs in the following order: for the lower central incisors between 6 and 7 years of age, lower lateral and upper central incisors between 7 and 8 years of age and for upper lateral incisors between 8 and 9 years of age. In addition, the eruption chronology used by the Paediatric Dentistry Department of the Faculty of Dentistry of the University of Chile is attached[1] (Table 6).

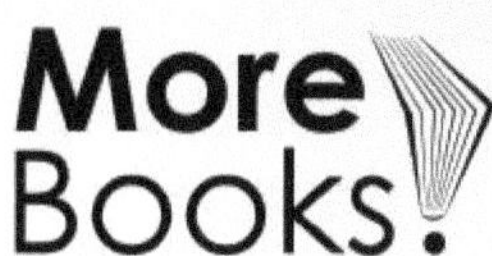

More
Books!

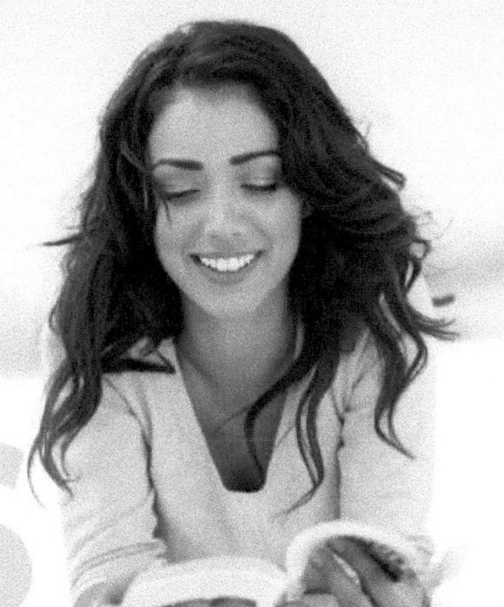

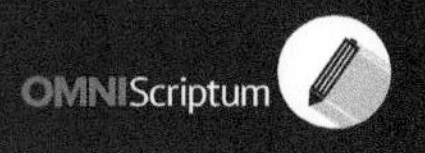

info@omniscriptum.com
www.omniscriptum.com
OMNIScriptum

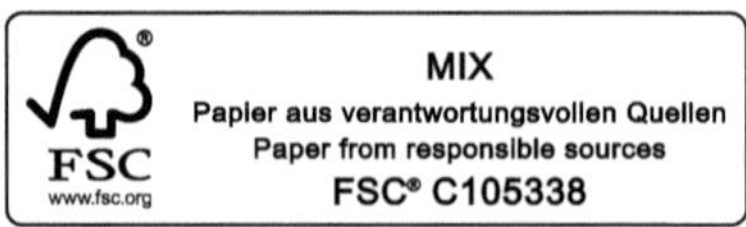

Printed by Books on Demand GmbH, Norderstedt / Germany